GERIATRIC DRUG USE— CLINICAL & SOCIAL PERSPECTIVES

Pergamon Titles of Related Interest

DiMatteo ACHIEVING PATIENT COMPLIANCE
Scientific International Research DRUG STUDIES IN CVD & PVD

Related Journals*

DRUG INFORMATION JOURNAL
EXPERIMENTAL GERONTOLOGY
INFORMATION SYSTEMS
INFORMATION PROCESSING AND MANAGEMENT
PHARMACEUTICAL AND BIOMEDICAL ANALYSIS

*Free specimen copies available upon request.

GERIATRIC DRUG USE– CLINICAL & SOCIAL PERSPECTIVES

Edited by

Steven R. Moore, RPh, MPH
Center for Drugs and Biologics
Food and Drug Administration
Rockville, MD

Thomas W. Teal, BS
Editor-in-Chief: DRUG INFORMATION JOURNAL
Director, Scientific Data Management
McNeil Pharmaceutical
Spring House, PA

The following are edited proceedings of the Drug Information
Association workshop "Geriatric Drug Use—Clinical and Social
Perspectives" held February 27 and 28, 1984 at the Sheraton
Washington Hotel, Washington, DC.

Pergamon Press
New York • Oxford • Paris • Frankfurt • Toronto • Sydney

RC
953.5
.G46
1985

Pergamon Press Offices:

U.S.A.   Pergamon Press Inc., Maxwell House, Fairview Park,
            Elmsford, New York 10523, U.S.A.

U.K.   Pergamon Press Ltd., Headington Hill Hall,
            Oxford OX3 0BW, England

CANADA   Pergamon Press Canada Ltd., Suite 104, 150 Consumers Road,
            Willowdale, Ontario M2J 1P9, Canada

AUSTRALIA   Pergamon Press (Aust.) Pty. Ltd., P.O. Box 544,
            Potts Point, NSW 2011, Australia

FRANCE   Pergamon Press SARL, 24 rue des Ecoles,
            75240 Paris, Cedex 05, France

FEDERAL REPUBLIC   Pergamon Press GmbH, Hammerweg 6,
OF GERMANY   D-6242 Kronberg-Taunus, Federal Republic of Germany

Copyright © 1985 Pergamon Press Inc.

Library of Congress Cataloging in Publication Data
Main entry under title:

Geriatric drug use.

    Proceedings of a Drug Information Association
workshop held Feb. 27-28, 1984, Washington, D.C.
    Includes index.
    1. Geriatric pharmacology--Congresses. 2. Drug
utilization--Congresses. I. Moore, Steven R.
II. Teal, Thomas W. III. Drug Information
Association. [DNLM: 1. Drug Therapy--in old age--
congresses. 2. Drug Utilization--congresses.
WT 100 G369   1984]
RC953.5.G46   1984   615.5′8′0880565   84-19011
ISBN 0-08-031939-4

Printed in the United States of America

CONTENTS

PART 7: RISK FACTORS IN GERIATRIC DRUG USE

PART 8: CLINICAL TESTING OF DRUGS IN THE ELDERLY

PART 9: HEALTH PROMOTION FOR THE ELDERLY

PART 10: INDUSTRY INVOLVEMENT IN GERIATRIC DRUG USE

PART 11: THE FUTURE IN GERIATRIC DRUG USE

PREFACE

In the field of public health, few areas offer the challenge accorded in the promotion of health among the elderly population. Beginning in May with Older Americans Month, the U.S. Public Health Service and the Administration on Aging are seeking to promote health among our elderly citizens. The theme, "Health: Make It Last a Lifetime," will be energetically promoted and the area of drug use among the elderly is one of the areas that will get top priority in this promotion.

In conjunction with this effort, the Drug Information Association brought together leaders in the field of geriatric drug use from government, academia, and industry to share the latest information related to all facets of the subject. The results of the meeting are presented here in the hope that the conclusions will stimulate further effort in the field.

C. Everett Koop, MD, ScD
Surgeon General
United States Public Health Service

Lennie-Marie P. Tolliver, PhD
Commissioner
Administration on Aging

PART 1

OPENING

Chapter 1

AN INTRODUCTION: CLINICAL PERSPECTIVES ON GERIATRIC DRUG USE

C. Everett Koop, MD, ScD

I am delighted to be introducing this collection of papers on drug usage among the elderly. It would be difficult to think of a more timely subject than this one to be addressed by the drug industry and the pharmacy and pharmacology professions. All the demographic, social, political, and bio-medical indicators tell us that the single most significant change in the character of American society is the growth of that segment of our population that is over the age of 65.

This book offers an excellent balance of concerns in the areas of social policy, patient care, biomedical research, and government-industry relations. A number of my colleagues representing these many concerns in the Department of Health and Human Services will be contributing. And I should add that, in the 3 years I've been Surgeon General, I've been impressed over and over again with the quality of leadership that is available to help attend to the social, physical, and mental health of our society. Good people are found throughout the U.S. Public Health Service and, indeed, throughout the Department of Health and Human Services itself.

Also, I've been pleased to see the degree to which the private sector has put forward its share of thoughtful, knowledgeable, and caring people who are also deeply concerned about the future course of our society. I know there are many questions in which government and the private sector disagree. And, much of the time, that's just the way it should be.

But I would say that where the issues are of consequence to the health status of our people, the public and the private sectors are not adversaries. Rather, they tend to put forward their best people to work together for what is good for our country. Our preference is clearly collaboration and consensus when it comes to the public health.

And this book is a good illustration of that. The contributors are top-notch. I say that not only because of the information they possess — which is considerable — but also for the commitment they've made to put their knowledge and experience to work for the benefit of our citizens, especially the most vulnerable of our citizens, the aging and the aged infirm.

Frankly, with the array of talent represented here, my role is not an easy one. Nevertheless, I do want to leave a message with you, something that may lend a larger public health perspective — or a context, if you will — to our deliberations. I mentioned the word "demography," but sheer numbers, as you well know, do not tell the whole story. If anything, the gross statistics — "one in five Americans," that sort of thing — screen off many significant demographic subsets.

For example, Dr Donald Custis, the former Chief Medical Director of the Veterans Administration, has been warning us that by 1990 about 60% of all men over the age of 65 will be veterans. If, at that time, veterans seek VA health care at the rate they are now seeking it, then, says Dr Custis, about 1.8 million veterans will be looking for VA care in 1990. But 10 years after that, in the year 2000, the figure will have climbed to 2.2 million veterans seeking VA care. They will be among the estimated 9 million veterans who will be among us by the turn of the century.

Each succeeding age cohort is more literate and better educated than the previous age cohort. All signs indicate that by the year 2000, our population of persons over age 65 will be more self-sufficient and more reachable — in terms of patient education — than any previous group. Today we are exhorting every American to take more personal responsibility for his or her health status. We're making some headway, but we'd like to be making more; and we will, as the years pass and the percentage grows of Americans who have the education and training to handle more personal health responsibility.

However, we are faced with so many unknowns in the field of health for the aging that we must be careful not to generalize too quickly or too often. All our projections are based upon life as we've known it so far, not life as it *will be* in the future. Let me give just one small example.

Over the past 15 years or so, there has been a virtual revolution in eye care and vision health among young adults and older working adults. As a result of this new concern with vision — that is, as a result of the many effective ways we treat diseases of the eye today and the many ways we prevent eye disease and injury from occurring — I believe we ought to rethink many of our programs for vision health. I think we will soon be able to do much more with the same resources we now have.

And other areas of public health for the aging are just now capturing our attention. For example, one major problem among the elderly is urinary incontinence. Some preliminary U.S. data seem to indicate that about one-half of all patients in nursing homes suffer from urinary incontinence. And if some British data are anywhere near the mark, another half million or so elderly suffer from urinary incontinence but are still living at home.

Incontinence can be a critical condition for tens of thousands of older people. It reduces their ability to live independent lives, it reduces their mobility, it is a humiliating condition and increases the potential for physical and social isolation. And incontinence can produce, of itself, other disease or disabling conditions, such as serious infections among catheterized patients.

Urinary incontinence can sometimes be a side effect from a prescription drug being taken for quite another purpose. A change of prescription, where possible, can solve the problem. Or the condition can be relieved or even reversed through surgery. But in other instances the solution may be in a combination of surgery, a drug, and new learned behavior. For instance, at the University of Michigan we are supporting research in combination behavior-and-drug therapy in clinical trials employing phenylpropanolamine and oxybutynin.

Behavior therapies hold out a great deal of hope for the incontinent elderly. As yet, however, we don't have a tested, clear idea of which therapies work and which ones do not. To help get that problem resolved, the National Institute on Aging, together with the NIH Division of Nursing, will soon be advertising a new round of grant proposals for behavioral therapies to reverse urinary incontinence.

We are talking about doing something to help a million or more older persons who are incontinent. It may not be as complicated or as dramatic a problem as heart disease, but it certainly affects the lives of at least as many people.

The Office of Surgeon General has taken a special interest in this problem and in one other, also a widespread but poorly understood problem of the elderly, osteoporosis, the loss of bone strength.

As with so many problems that affect the health of older people, we have suspicions about how important and far-reaching the problem of osteoporosis may be, but we have very little reliable, hard data to go on. Some experts say that as many as 15 million Americans suffer from osteoporosis, but — absent a tight and generally acceptable definition of "osteoporosis" — such numbers are not reliable. And the disease itself is not thoroughly understood. Hence, there is as yet no accepted, safe, effective treatment for osteoporosis. Nevertheless, as little as we know, we still know enough to feel we must move ahead and do what is possible.

The second issue I would call to your attention is hip fractures. An estimated 200,000 hip fractures occur each year among persons of all ages. Of course, the great majority of fractures occur among the elderly: The typical age among persons reported to have had a hip fracture is in the mid to late 70s.

But the nature of the event is not clear. Does a person fall down and fracture the hip, which is the common notion, or does a person fracture a hip and then fall down, which is the sequence I believe is more typical? As yet, we don't know the answer. Is it important? Very much so.

At least one of every four hip fractures causes in some way the death of the person with that fracture, usually within 1 year. It is a contributing factor to the deaths of many more persons. Current estimates put the total at about 35,000 premature deaths each year, a considerable number. According to other data, almost as many victims — another 26,000 — go on living but can no longer walk. They represent an enormous burden to their families, their communities, and to themselves.

It seems quite clear in just these two areas alone — urinary incontinence and osteoporosis — that we can save many thousands of lives and many millions of dollars with well-placed investments of time, interest, and money. And those are the kinds of investments we are making. I have concentrated on these two areas because they represent not only the possibilities of our gaining new biomedical knowledge, but they also are among the costliest conditions affecting the nation's elderly: Incontinence and hip fractures cost Medicare alone in excess of $2 billion each year.

There is so much public distress at the high cost of care for the elderly that I am truly concerned about our country maintaining its political will to support this kind of insurance. A great deal of thought and effort is going into research and demonstration programs that tinker with the funding and the reimbursement mechanisms. And all that is important, to be sure. But to my way of thinking, the real solution will come when we have the means to control, reverse, or prevent the major, more costly disease and disability conditions of older people.

Readers of this volume will be hearing from Dr T. Franklin Williams, the Director of the NIA and a strong supporter of all the research initiatives that hold out hope for the aging. His agenda, of course, is central to many of your individual interests, I am sure. I have great respect for him and his staff and I am sure you will feel as encouraged as I do, once you have read his message.

But let me offer this word of caution to those of you who would focus on the disease conditions of the elderly *to the exclusion of* the health concerns of all other age groups: You can't do it. It just doesn't work. We have become so specialized in medicine, as in so many other things, that we sometimes truly believe that human growth moves from one neat little category to the next: One day we are known as "infants," the next, we are in early childhood, then, prepubescence, followed by adolescence and young adulthood. Then we are "working adults," as opposed to the other kind, who are fortunate enough not to have a category of their own.

And then, of course, we become "older people" and the "aged."

It is certainly a handy way to deal with the normal life span. But this kind of pigeonholing tends to give the impression that health problems occur for the individual — almost spontaneously — as soon as he or she leaves one category and enters the next one. And that's just not so.

The fact of the matter is that many disease conditions of the elderly can be traced to the kind of care they received as infants — in their diet and their immunization records as children. Many young people suffer trauma on the highway or in sports, and we know that the effects linger and become aggravated as old age sets in. The stress of a bad marriage, the effects of being an abused child and an abusing parent, alcoholism, drug abuse — all these and many, many other conditions of the body, the mind, and the spirit, experienced early in life, have profound effects on the individual as she or he enters the fifth and sixth decades.

How much better off many of our older persons would be, if, as adolescents, they had been exposed to — and had taken seriously — the kind of health promotion and disease prevention message that today is carried far and wide by virtually every responsible health agency, public or private. The toll taken by tobacco alone — the lung and heart and gastrointestinal diseases generated by cigarette smoking — that toll would not be suffered by millions of Americans and their families.

And the terrible damage from alcohol — not just the collapse of diseased internal organs, but the interpersonal damage, the homicides, and the family violence that so frequently accompany alcohol — that damage would not be borne by so many of our elderly if they had been impressed in their youth with the dangers of heavy drinking.

And the weak bones and muscle groups, the loss of teeth, the gastrointestinal diseases, the blunting of many mental processes, all these and other phenomena might occur with much less frequency or intensity — or not at all — had the individual paid closer attention to his or her daily nutritional needs.

The same can be said of such behaviors as compliance, or following directions for taking medicines. So many physicians have told me that one of the most discouraging aspects of treating the elderly is their cavalier attitude toward the regimens for drug-taking. Many elderly patients don't fill the prescriptions they are given. Others fill but then ignore them, or they get refills of medicines that have become favorites but are no longer safe and effective for their condition.

Some older patients obtain prescriptions — quite legally — from two or three different physicians who are often unknown to each other, and may therefore be getting drugs that ought not be taken together. Still others fill prescriptions and then decide for themselves what the regimen should be — how much to take and when to take it.

Of course, some older people respond this way because they feel financial pressure and try to cut a corner here or there — including the medicine corner. No, I'm talking about the older person who, in earlier years, had little experience with — or respect for — pharmaceuticals and has not changed, even though life itself can be riding on the proper use of these drugs.

We are fairly positive that one of the best behaviors an older person can cultivate is that of being aware of his or her own body — what it is doing and how it is doing it. We are asking our research populations to adopt this behavior, but for many of them it is new, uncomfortable, and strange. They've had a lifetime of being unconcerned about their personal health and disrespectful of their own bodies, and some of them, whether correctly or not, feel it is simply too late to reverse themselves and learn a new and more sensible kind of personal health behavior.

I will close my introduction with this single but sincere plea:

> Do not look upon the problems of geriatric health — including drug usage — as isolated in any way from health problems affecting the entire life span. They are not. One's life evolves within a seamless web of circumstance. Compartmentalization may be intellectually desirable, but it is biologically untenable. I believe that effective medical care should benefit not only today's elderly — who are very much on our minds in this context — but also today's children, youth, and young adults — *tomorrow's* elderly.

That smacks a little of those lines from one of the earliest treatises written on the subject of old age. Cicero was the author, more than 2,000 years ago. He himself was murdered in Rome, poor man, at the age of 63 and never got to enjoy what he believed would be a wonderful time of life. He said:

> Give me a young man in whom there is something of the old, and an old man with something of the young: guided so, a man may grow old in body but never in the mind.

I think he was absolutely right.

Chapter 2

SOCIAL PERSPECTIVES ON GERIATRIC DRUG USE

Lennie-Marie P. Tolliver, PhD

Given the reduced mortality, increased longevity, and the low birth rate of the population we are rapidly becoming an aging society. One in every nine Americans is 65 years of age or older and every day more than 1,000 people reach age 65. Today about 25 million Americans are 65 years and older, about 11% of our people. By the year 2030 the elderly population will include 55 million people, or about 18% of our total population. Within this group of older people the proportion of persons aged 65 to 74 is shrinking while the group of persons 75 and older is growing. It is anticipated that this trend will continue until at least the end of this century.

These are very significant demographic changes in relation to drug utilization. The aging of the population, especially the growth in the 75 and older age group, means a potential increase in the incidence of chronic illness and disabilities. Such an increase in disease and impairments may result in a growing use of over-the-counter and prescription drugs and thus increase the likelihood of a greater incidence of drug misuse and abuse, adverse reactions, and drug interactions.

The clinical aspects of geriatric drug use are enormously important to consider so that potential drug problems can be avoided in dealing with older people. However, other factors can also impact on the older person increasing the risk of such problems in this group. The social reality in which a person lives can exert a strong influence on the way drugs are used. For example, with the tendency toward increased mobility of family members, geographical distances hamper the care-taking role of the family elderly. Today many elderly people live quite some distance from their children. Although many older persons prefer to live alone, living by oneself means that there is no one to remind the older person to take a drug, to help ensure that instructions are followed, or to notice when problems start to occur.

Another factor that can adversely affect the elderly is the prevalent notion that drugs are a no-risk cure. The dangers of older people using over-the-counter drugs, especially in combination with prescription drugs, have been widely discussed.

Still another issue involves mistaken notions about older people and the aging process itself. Erroneous assumptions that aging is synonymous with disease can lead to over- or under-medicating elderly patients. Adverse drug reactions can be missed if symptoms are dismissed as "senility" when, in fact, confusion, memory loss, and disorientation may be the side effects of drugs.

The very nature of the complex health care delivery system of today, so totally different than 50 or even 25 years ago, is still another social reality that can create problems for older people. Technologically sophisticated and functionally specialized, the health care system today is one in which there is rarely a single service provider who coordinates all aspects of a patient's health care. Rather, there are several providers, each with a specific focus. In such a system, responsibility for coordinating and monitoring overall care rests with the patient. Horror stories abound of overdosage and drug interactions due to drugs being prescribed by different physicians or poor communication between the patient and the physician.

The drug delivery system can also be a factor influencing drug problems of the elderly. For example, drug packaging can create problems for older persons. Although "child-proof" safety caps on medication bottles are very important to protect youngsters, older people with arthritic fingers cannot negotiate the mechanics of such caps. Inability to get the drug out of a bottle can cause noncompliance among the elderly.

Other noncompliance problems include over- or underuse of drugs that occurs when older people forget whether or not they have taken their medicine and either take an extra dose or omit a dose. The lack of appropriate consumer education relating to geriatric drug use contributes to improper uses of drugs such as failure to follow time, amount, or dietary requirements accompanying the use of a drug; incorrect storage; use of outdated drugs; sharing or borrowing of drugs; and failure to monitor or report side effects. It has even been documented that failure of older persons to follow prescribed drug dosages can lead to such tragic outcomes as habituation and suicide.

Although certainly not all-inclusive, the factors I have mentioned can and do cause serious drug problems for older people. Health professionals have a vital role to play in reducing the incidence of drug misuse and helping older people benefit from appropriate use of medications. The role of the physician in this regard is pivotal. Patient-physician communication is critical to the appropriate use of drugs by the elderly. Physicians need to devote enough time to older people to give them instructions about drugs and how and when to take them. Communication must be clear and in language that older patients can understand. Thorough knowledge of the drugs an older person might be taking must be elicited so that monitoring of the elderly patient's drug use can be effective.

Like the physician, the pharmacist has a critical role to play in assuring the safe and effective use of prescription and over-the-counter drugs among the elderly. During the last decade, clinically trained pharmacists have significantly expanded their patient care responsibilities to the elderly, including assessment of drug response, identification of drug-induced adverse effects and drug interactions, and drug compliance through patient education.

Other specific strategies for health professionals that can reduce noncompliance with drug regimens among older people relate to removing, or at least reducing, barriers to safe and effective drug use. For example, a significant number of the elderly suffer from hearing loss. The communication barrier due to hearing loss can be reduced by determining the amount of loss and accommodating for it. Visual loss can be countered by using large letters, boldface type, and large labels for written materials. Also effective may be the use of a color-coding system in which a colored dot is placed on each medication container and a corresponding dot of the same color is placed on a medication calendar at the time the medication is to be administered. Medication calendars are also useful to help older people accommodate for memory loss. Patients with dexterity problems can be helped if health professionals advise the elderly of the availability of non-child-resistant medication containers.

Physicians and pharmacists can reduce risk factors related to complex drug regimens by placing the name and purpose of each medication on the container. Such labeling should be simple, direct, and in terminology easily understood by elderly patients, for example, "Digoxin — heart pill"; "Ampicillin — antibiotic for infection"; and "Lasix — water pill." Another approach to reducing risk factors related to problems of complex regimens includes the use of a patient profile system, which may help prevent noncompliance and drug interactions resulting from a polypharmacy situation. For those elderly patients living with or near relatives, every effort should be made to involve these family members in the compliance-improving strategy.

These are some of the ways in which today's health professionals can and are implementing flexible approaches to serving a constantly growing older population. At the federal level, the Department of Health and Human Services is supporting a number of initiatives that seek to reduce drug misuse among older people and enhance the benefits of appropriate drug regimens. The Administration on Aging (AoA), for example, supports 11 Long-Term Care Gerontology Centers across the country. Among other undertakings, the centers have developed, implemented, and supported demonstrations, research, education, training, and public information programs that seek to improve geriatric drug use. AoA also supports the Aging Health Policy Center at the University of California in San Francisco, which recently developed a major policy paper on drugs and the elderly.

In addition, AoA has joined with the Public Health Service in cooperative support of a National Health Promotion Initiative for Older People. Drug use and misuse is one of the four areas targeted for specific activities by our agencies.

At other levels, in both the public and private sectors, initiatives have been implemented to address the problems of drug misuse, especially among older people. For example, computer-based drug monitoring systems have been developed in order to detect potential adverse drug reactions, including drug interactions. These systems maintain a patient profile that includes all medicines a patient has taken over a specified period of time. Such systems are already in use by a number of chain drug stores and pharmacies, hospitals, and health maintenance organizations.

The National Voluntary Organizations for Independent Living for the Aging (NVOILA) has a grant from AoA to stimulate its more than 200 members to carry out a variety of activities for the aging. The American Pharmaceutical Association (APhA) and the National Pharmaceutical Council (NPC) are two members of NVOILA who have launched major activities to improve drug use by older persons. For example, the American Pharmaceutical Association (APhA), in cooperation with the American Red Cross, designed a form that helps older people keep track of their drug regimens on a daily basis. In addition to providing older people with these forms, the Red Cross utilizes them for teaching purposes in classes they run for care givers of frail and impaired older people.

APhA also developed several educational programs that have been used by state associations and schools of pharmacy for professional and continuing-education purposes. They have also been used by individual pharmacists who volunteer their time to educate groups of older consumers.

The National Pharmaceutical Council operates state-level conference programs designed to identify unmet needs and information gaps in both professional and consumer spheres of concern. Follow-up activities include the planning of initiatives designed to meet those information gaps and other needs identified at the conferences.

The council also developed and runs an ongoing project in Texas, Massachusetts, and Rhode Island, with two more states expected to participate this year. The project, called the Brown Bag Program, brings pharmacists, pharmacy students, senior citizens organizations, church groups, state and area agencies on aging staff, nutrition site staff and participants, and senior centers staff and participants together in cooperative partnerships to provide direct consumer education to the elderly. Older people are invited to put all their medications, including both over-the-counter and prescription drugs, into a bag and bring them to predesignated sites. At these sites pharmacists and pharmacy students review all the drugs the older person has brought in and then advises the person about any possible drug interactions, side effects, outdated medications, and the like, providing the counseling the older person needs in order to reduce drug mishaps and assure the benefits of an appropriate drug regimen.

State and area agencies on aging across the country have implemented numerous activities designed to help older people utilize medications appropriately and avoid drug problems. Some of these undertakings, to cite just a few, include the training of area agency personnel in Vermont, Michigan, South Carolina, and Tennessee. Training programs address drug use, misuse, and methods to reduce drug problems among older people. The State Agency on Aging in New Hampshire has set up speaker bureaus for a statewide drug education program for the elderly. The Division on Aging in New Jersey funded a contract with the New Jersey Pharmaceutical Association to develop an eight-county program to train retired pharmacists to counsel groups of older people about drugs. All 15 of Kentucky's area agencies are participating in a program that seeks to reduce drug misuse by older persons, and Arkansas has a Brown Bag Program similar to the one I described in Texas, Massachusetts, and Rhode Island. In Oklahoma the State Agency on Aging supported training for all state and area agency on aging staff concerning drug use and misuse among older people, and, of the 11 Area Agencies on Aging in Oklahoma, 8 have various types of programs dealing with older peoples' problems related to drug misuse, and the others are now reviewing similar projects. These are only several examples of ongoing initiatives implemented and supported by aging agencies across the nation in the area of geriatric drug use.

Other activities concerned with consumer education of the elderly about drug use have also been implemented around the country in recent years and are designed specifically to improve the understanding of older people about the drugs they take. These programs may serve as models for the development of other projects. Some of these include:

- The Elder-Ed Program at the University of Maryland, where retired pharmacists are paired with pharmacy students to provide consumer drug education to older people at a variety of locations, such as senior centers, senior citizen apartments, churches, and synagogues

- The Senior Medication Program in San Francisco, which utilizes a number of pharmacies as health information centers for older people — in areas with heavy concentrations of older people with language barriers drug information was displayed in several languages in the participating pharmacies. (In 1980, the program was integrated into the San Francisco Department of Public Health and now serves as a model for a joint undertaking involving private and public funding sources.)

- An effective grass-roots effort at drug education for seniors called Connexion, Inc, in Flint, Michigan — Connexion is an affiliate agency of the Genesee County Commission on Substance Abuse Services and the Genesee

County Pharmaceutical Association. (The program began in 1978 when the county Pharmaceutical Association combined efforts with Connexion, Inc, and began outreach instruction about the proper and safe use of medications at senior citizen nutrition sites and apartment complexes.)

From the examples I have outlined it is clear that there are a number of approaches that can be utilized to solve problems of drug misuse and abuse among the elderly and assure that older people receive the maximum benefit from appropriate drug regimens. Leadership can be exercised by health professionals, organizations, agencies, and communities to encourage innovative programs for the education of older consumers and their care givers as well as professional and continuing education for practitioners and service providers regarding the clinical and social aspects of geriatric drug use. As the aging population of our country continues to increase, it is essential that present and future health care practitioners and others who work with the elderly are equipped with the educational tools they *need* to provide older Americans with the health care they *deserve*.

BIBLIOGRAPHY

Lee PR, Lipton HL: *Drugs and the Elderly*. Policy paper No. 3. San Francisco, Aging Health Policy Center, University of California at San Francisco, 1983.

Luedke SM, Reese SS: Drug use and abuse among the elderly, in Oliver DB, Foster CA, Whitney KN (eds): *Human Responses to Aging — Therapy and Practice*. San Antonio, TX, Trinity University, 1976.

Wise Drug Use for the Elderly. Washington, DC, Center for Human Services, 1979.

PART 2

INFLUENCING THE ELDERLY DRUG USER AND PROVIDER

Chapter 3

ISSUES IN GERIATRIC LABELING REVISIONS

Lloyd G. Millstein, PhD

In 1956, Dr Louis Lasagna summarized knowledge of how drug effects are modified by aging and concluded that "what is obviously required is a good deal more work and a good deal less talk."[1] In the quarter century that has passed since that statement, some important strides have been made; however, we are just now at the proverbial "cutting edge."

One of the attempts by the Food and Drug Administration has been in the labeling of prescription drugs to provide to the health professional guidance in treating the elderly. In 1979, the FDA published a regulation[2] revising the format and providing new content for labeling of prescription drugs. This regulation brought up to date the previous regulation, which dated back to 1938. This well-defined format provides the prescriber with the information he or she will need to ensure proper use of the individual drug, even in the case of special populations — for example, the elderly patient. Although no specific section heading is designated for the elderly patient as it currently is for the pediatric patient, information for the elderly is often included in the sections entitled pharmacokinetics, special situations of use, contraindications, warnings, precautions, adverse reactions, and dosage and administration. In some cases this information is highlighted specifically for the elderly patient. For example:

Indications and Usage section

If evidence is available to support the safety and effectiveness of the drug only in selected subgroups of the larger population with a disease . . . eg, patients with mild disease or patients in a special age group . . . .

Contraindications section

. . . Those situations in which the drug should not be used because the risk of use clearly outweighs any possible benefit. These situations include adminis-

tration of the drug to patients . . . because of their age . . . have a substantial
risk of being harmed by it.

Dosage and Administration section
   . . . any modification of dosage needed in special patient populations, eg,
. . . in geriatric age groups . . . .

Drug manufacturers have been encouraged to include this information
when it is based on clinical evaluations of their drug in patients over the age
of 65 years, because, even with the most carefully planned medical care, elderly patients are more prone than younger patients to develop adverse reactions to drugs or to respond in an unexpected manner.[3]

The purpose of this paper is to discuss how drug information for the elderly
may be presented using the current labeling format and to present also a new
proposed section specifically devoted to geriatric information.

Because drugs in the older individual frequently produce a more profound
and longer-lasting pharmacological response than the same dose given to a
younger person, information should be presented on the four areas of pharmacokinetics — absorption, distribution, metabolism, and excretion. Limited
information at this time indicates that drug absorption is not appreciably
altered in old age.[4,5] However, the decreased intestinal blood flow that accompanies the physiological changes in the elderly might be expected to have
an effect on absorption. In addition, the large number of drugs taken by
the elderly, averaging more than 13 prescriptions per year[5] including renew-
als, would indicate potential interference with proper or optimum absorption, especially for those drugs that alter gastric and small intestinal motility
— for example, anticholinergics and opiates. Conversely, other drugs such
as laxatives shorten intestinal transit time.

Inappropriate and incorrect use of drugs in the elderly is reflected in a
higher percentage of untoward effects.[6] Most are identified readily when single drugs are given and no more than a single disease is present to confound
the evaluation. Many reactions are lost in the induced disturbances of physiologic balance that occur more readily in the aged. Improper dosage, inju-
dicious methods of administration, and lack of awareness of drug interactions
are common and are often associated with failure to quantitate the reactive
capacities of aging body resources. The fact that aging alters drug effects
and that drug actions alter senescent functions emphasizes the need to be
familiar with the roster of confirmed pharmacologic data. Improved treatment of the individual would result from such observance. Medication schedules must be in line with recognized levels of normality in aging. These
precautions will reduce the chances of initiating primary or sequential mishaps when drugs are administered to the elderly who are more susceptible
to side effects and less likely to be responsive to reparative measures.[6]

To more clearly focus on the needs of the elderly, and to provide the
prescriber with meaningful guidance, the Division of Drug Advertising and

Labeling will be proposing the inclusion of a section in the prescription drug labeling regulations on geriatric use. The proposed statement reads:

> Geriatric Use: A specific geriatric indication, if any, shall be described under the 'Indications and Usage' section of the labeling, and appropriate dosage for elderly patients shall be stated under the 'Dosage and Administration' section of the labeling.
>
> If use of a drug in the elderly is associated with a specific hazard, the hazard shall be described in this subsection of the labeling or in the section of the labeling considered to be most appropriate due to degree of risk or subject matter, eg, drug interaction or laboratory test that should be observed because of drug specificity of action in the elderly; and this subsection of the labeling shall refer to it.

This is a signal to the drug industry to begin the examination of clinical data for patients over the age of 65 for patterns that need the specific attention of the prescriber. What we are looking for and what companies have started to do is to separate the clinical and adverse responses in elderly patients during a clinical trial. If the response to the drug was significantly different in the elderly as opposed to those patients under 65 or 75, then this should be stated. If the side effect profile is clearly different in the older patient then this should be so stated. If the dosage required to obtain optimum response is different, this should be clearly stated. Because of the usual presence of other medications in the elderly population, diuretics, beta- and calcium-blockers, antihypertensives, antiarthritic agents, and the array of OTC products (laxatives, pain killers, antacids), careful examination of drug interactions is crucial to care in this population.

Based mainly on the FDA proposed guidelines for testing drugs in the elderly patient, there are nine rules that must be adhered to.

1. No exclusion from clinical trials because of age — at least during Phase III testing

2. Consider specific age-related changes in pharmacokinetics or pharmacodynamics

3. Examination of responses by elderly subjects and/or patients in clinical studies — separation of beneficial effects and adverse effects by dose

4. Drugs excreted by the kidneys need examination in patients with various degrees of kidney malfunction

5. Information for dosing instructions that provides adjustments for renal impairment

6. Labeling to include means of calculating creatinine clearance from the serum creatinine, adjusting for weight and age

7. Examination of the precise pattern of metabolism in the elderly including the minor pathways of metabolism

8. Drug interactions to be anticipated from protein binding; interaction with drugs commonly used by the elderly

9. Special consideration, if necessary, for the elderly female

Table 3.1 shows examples of the physiological changes associated with aging that have been observed over the past years and are just now having an impact on labeling changes.[5] This is important for prescribers to be aware of and important for the drug industry to examine in the development of their own drug entities.

Table 3.1. Physiological Changes Associated With Aging — Impact On Labeling

System	Changes with Aging
Cardiovascular	Cardiac output after age 80: 70% of that at age 30; decreased contractile force and cardiac reserve; decrease of 8% in plasma volume from age 20 to 80
Endocrine	Decrease in estrogen and testosterone; response to glucose tolerance test more prolonged with slow return to normal
Musculoskeletal	Decrease of 17% in lean body mass and total body water from age 20 to 80; osteoporosis; bony sclerosis
Gastrointestinal	Decreased peristalsis; reduced gastric acid secretion and intestinal blood flow
Genitourinary	Decline in glomerular filtration rate; BUN rises to 15–20 mg%
Integumentary	Decreased activity of sebaceous glands; loss of subcutaneous tissue; pigmentary changes in skin with thinning; loss of elasticity
Nervous	Organic deteriorations
Respiratory	Loss of functional units in the lung
Body as a whole	Increase of 35% in body fat as proportion of body weight from age 20 to 70; slower and less vigorous response from immune system; decrease in total body potassium; less caloric requirements and greater vitamin needs

Finally, as a result of the labeling format revision program, I want to show examples of the kinds of changes that are appearing and will be appearing more frequently in labeling in the future.

Antihistamines: *Warnings* section
Use in the elderly (approximately 60 years or older): Antihistamines are more likely to cause dizziness, sedation, and hypotension in elderly patients.

Phenothiazines: *Clinical Pharmacology* section
Age is considered an important determinant of the rates of metabolism and excretion of the phenothiazines. The elderly, the fetus, and the infant have diminished capacities to metabolize and excrete these drugs.

Cholecystographic agents: *Warnings* section
Cholecystography in elderly, severely ill, or debilitated patients may result in renal shut down.

Warfarin sodium: *Precautions* section
Special risk patients: Caution should be observed when warfarin sodium is administered to certain patients such as the elderly or debilitated.

Research has shown that there is a wide range of differences in drug responses from person to person, more so from age 65 to advanced senescence. However, there are regular and assessable changes with aging that can be applied to geriatric therapeutics[6,7]; these are:

1. The selection of drugs least likely to induce untoward effects is a significant precaution in the administration of the initial and subsequent doses, particularly those with cumulative tendencies.

2. Forms of administration (dose, route, frequency), as well as concern for physical and chemical imbalances, may need adjusting for the aging decline in physiology.

3. Combinations of drugs may interact with the displacement of one or more from their conjugated state in a way that can precipitate an unexpected and untoward chain of events.

4. Identification must be made of the fine line between the normal body limitations of aging that increase susceptibility to drugs and the nature of the pathologic condition for which the medication is required that may heighten the possibilities of adverse results.

We are once again on the threshold of change for professional labeling — this time to benefit the group long overdue for some benefit, the elderly. We now know the direction, and it is time to more forward.

REFERENCES

1. Lasagna L: Drug effects as modified by aging. *Proc Assoc Res Nerv Ment Dis* 1956; 35:83.

2. Content and format for labeling of human prescription drugs. *Federal Register* June 26, 1979; 44:37434.

3. Williamson J: Prescribing problems in the elderly. *Practitioner* 1978; 220:749.

4. Drugs in the elderly, editorial. *Br Med J* May 6, 1978; 1:1168.

5. Vestal RE: Designing therapy for the elderly. *Drugs and the Elderly* NIA Science Writer Seminar Series, DHEW Publication No. (NIH) 78-1449. Washington, DC, DHEW, 1978; 9:49.

6. Kenny AD: Designing therapy for the elderly. *Drug Therapy* July, 1979; 9:49.

7. Freeman JT: Some principles of medication in geriatrics. *J. Am Geriatr Soc* 1974; 22:289.

Chapter 4

PHARMACY INTERVENTIONS

Nancy J. Olins, MA

This chapter will discuss strategies for influencing the elderly medication user and provider and, specifically, interventions focusing on pharmacy. Generally, the literature is scant and this is an area that has been neglected as a potential focus for provider and user education.

Four areas affecting the older consumer of medications will be covered. First, findings of two Food and Drug Administration studies will be reviewed and summarized, arguing a need for improved or reinforced drug information and education. Second, some ongoing federal, local, and private sector interventions attempting to influence the elderly will be reviewed. Third, experiences of the American Association of Retired Persons (AARP) Pharmacy Service with our own prescription drug information program geared to the elderly will be provided. The chapter will end with some thoughts for future studies.

One thousand one office-based physicians and dispensing pharmacists were questioned about patient information and prescription drugs in a telephone survey by Louis Harris and Associates for an FDA study. The compilation of data reflects that:

- Physicians feel patients are satisfied with the information they're receiving because few questions are asked by patients,

- Seventy-nine percent of physicians say they spend sufficient time informing patients about drugs through a variety of written and visual materials. In fact, 37% say they distribute materials they have prepared themselves,

- Physicians are quite satisfied with their own efforts to inform and educate their patients about the proper use of prescription drugs,

- Pharmacists say they are asked questions with one out of every three prescriptions they fill,

- Eighty-two percent of pharmacists do think patients should ask more questions.

However, when patients are surveyed, as done by Chilton Research for FDA, the findings differ radically from those of Harris and Associates.

Next, a national survey measured patient receipt of prescription drug information. This was a randomized study of 1,104 patients who had received a new prescription within the previous 4 weeks.

- Only 2% to 4% of patients say they asked questions about their prescriptions while in the physician's office,

- Six percent of patients report receiving any written information from their doctors,

- Only 3% of patients report asking their pharmacists how much medicine to take, when to take it, information on refills, precautions, or side effects,

- Fifteen percent report receiving any written information in the pharmacy,

- Younger patients were three times more likely to ask questions about taking medications than older patients,

- Respondents over 60 (16% of the population) were half as likely to be counseled about directions for using medications as younger patients.

These two surveys highlight some glaring problems of communication between physicians and patients, and pharmacists and patients. They argue for interventions of all types to increase patient understanding, awareness, and compliance.

It is well established that the elderly comprise 11% of the population yet consume around 25% to 30% of all prescriptions. These Harris and Chilton results therefore take on an added significance. There *are* communication problems between patients and providers: Patients do not ask questions and this is a particular problem among the elderly. Estimates of prescription noncompliance range from 25% to 60%. While this number may be comparable to the general adult population, it is compounded among the elderly, who have numerous chronic diseases and purchase approximately 20 prescriptions per year.

What types of interventions are being attempted by pharmacists? I will review some current federally funded studies by the National Institute on Aging (NIA) and the National Center for Health Services Research (NCHSR), as well as some private sector activities.

NIA, under its small grant pilot studies, awarded a 1-year grant to Tyson Gibbs, MD, of Meharry Medical College. The design is a pharmacy-based study of the relation between pharmacy personnel and patients and compares advice-seeking activities of people between ages 18 and 64 to those over age 65. The outcome will determine the influence of patient age on advice-seeking compliance; and determine whether or not the elderly follow the advice they receive from pharmacy personnel at a rate different from other age groups. Results are expected in December 1984.

In 1979, NCHSR began a grant program to encourage research on improving the quality and economy of prescription drug use. Three projects are relevant.

The first is a study by Dr Francis Palumbo of the University of Maryland School of Pharmacy. His study is being conducted at 35 nursing homes in the Baltimore-Washington area and involves 540 patients. The study is aimed at improving the quality of drug use in nursing homes, and interventions include providing feedback to physicians on their own prescribing and educational materials for nurses. Outcomes include improvements in geriatric drug prescribing and drug administration. Data are now being analyzed and a final report is expected by early 1985.

Next is a 5-year grant to William Schaffner, MD, of Vanderbilt University for a controlled experiment of educational interventions to improve prescribing practices among physicians. Activities include written brochures, visits by physicians, and pharmacist visits. The study focuses on physician prescribing. Findings show that more cautious prescribing can improve quality and reduce costs of care. The medications studied were antibiotics, psychotropic drugs, and propoxyphene. At this time, field analysis is being performed. The grant is scheduled to be completed towards the end of 1984. The elderly, although included in the Medicaid population, are not the primary focus of this study.

Another educational intervention study supported by NCHSR was awarded to Jerry Avorn, MD, at the Harvard Medical School Division on Aging. Dr Avorn describes his study in chapter 12. This 3-year study was completed in 1982. Dr Avorn ran a controlled trial of medical school "detailing" with the goals of informing physicians of the ineffectiveness of certain widely used drugs and recommending more useful, as well as less expensive, alternatives. They used "unadvertisements" that looked like drug promotional materials followed up by pharmacist visits.

Examples of other educational efforts are the Elder-Ed and Elder-Health Programs at the University of Maryland School of Pharmacy. Through Elder-Ed, retired pharmacists are paired with pharmacy students to provide drug education to the elderly at neighborhood senior centers, apartment complexes, and health fairs. Major program objectives include the effective and safe use of medications, prevention of misuse of drugs, and involvement of the elderly in their own health care.

Because many elderly are not reached through Elder-Ed, a second educational program was developed — Elder-Health. Through this program faculty, students, and retired pharmacists train the care givers — visiting nurses, social workers, and family members — to provide services and information to the elderly in various settings.

On a local level, the city of San Francisco's Department of Health has been involved in educational interventions for the elderly. Their SRx program (which stands for Senior's Medication Education Program) focuses on improving the health of the elderly through information on the safe, rational use of medications. The program is staffed by health educators, graduate pharmacy students, and pharmacists. No evaluation has been conducted, so it is difficult to assess which component of the program is most significant.

Pharmacist interventions can also be seen in the nursing home setting. Medicare and Medicaid regulations require monthly drug regimen reviews in skilled nursing facilities and intermediate care facilities. According to the regulations, pharmacists review charts to protect the patient from nonessential drug therapy and current or evolving adverse drug effects. Pharmacists review PRN orders and validate that orders have been followed. The aim is to eliminate unnecessary or potentially harmful drugs and to reduce unneeded lab procedures.

These activities are very fragmented and there is a diverse array of pharmacy-based programs in nursing home settings. Only a handful have been designed to permit any evaluation of their impact. No consensus has emerged concerning efficacy and proper design.

We at the AARP Pharmacy Service became involved in providing prescription drug information to our 16 million members about 3 years ago and were the first group to distribute written prescription drug information to consumers when they receive their medications.

To provide some background, the AARP Pharmacy Service provides prescription and nonprescription and other health care items to AARP members. We are a nonprofit service filling more than 6 million prescriptions per year through eight regional mail-service pharmacy centers and two walk-in facilities. We have been in existence for 25 years and as of this year have filled 70 million prescriptions. We are the largest private mail service pharmacy in the world, serving millions of AARP members.

We began providing written drug information because approximately 90% of the prescriptions we fill are delivered by mail or other delivery service. Having a reference binder or book available on a pharmacy counter is of very little benefit to many of the elderly who do not pick up their medicines in person.

When we started this program, we distributed five leaflets. We are now distributing 59 separate drug leaflets, representing over 200 drugs. To date, over 4 million Medication Information Leaflets for Seniors (MILS) have been printed and nearly 3.5 million MILS have been sent to AARP members.

The MILS, prepared in conjunction with FDA and experts in geriatric medicine and pharmacy, tell in easy-to-understand language the various names of a medication, what conditions to take it for, how it should be taken, possible side effects, food and alcohol interactions, and information that patients should tell their doctor before taking the drug. One of our biggest concerns is that the print size be large with a lot of white space and clear graphics. See Figure 4.1(a-f) for a sample MILS.

25

Important Information about You and your Medication...

Thiazide and Related Drugs

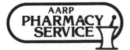

Provided by AARP Pharmacy Service,
with the assistance and cooperation of
the U.S. Food and Drug Administration,
and experts in geriatric medicine and
pharmacy.

Figure 4.1a. Sample Medication Information Leaflet for Seniors (MILS).

Name of your medication:
Thiazide and Related Drugs

Other names:
Hydrochlorothiazide (Hydrodiuril, Esidrix), Chlorothiazide (Diuril), Chlorthalidone (Hygroton).

What is it?
They are diuretics or water pills.

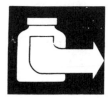

What is it for?

- They are used to lower high blood pressure.
- Thiazide drugs help the body get rid of extra salt and water due to heart, liver or kidney disease.

How long will you have to take it?

- Probably for the rest of your life.
- This medicine cannot cure high blood pressure, but if taken as directed, can help control it.

Figure 4.1b. Sample MILS, page 2.

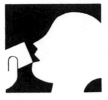

How should you take this medication?

- Take as directed, preferably in the morning after breakfast.
- Try to take every day at the same time.
- If you take two doses a day, take the second one in the evening before dinner.
- Do not take two doses at the same time.
- If you forget to take the first dose, take only your usual second dose.
- Do not take after dinner. It may interrupt your sleep and cause you to urinate (pass water).
- Do NOT stop taking if you feel better.

Things to remember:

- Do not rise quickly after lying down or sitting. You may feel dizzy or lightheaded.

Figure 4.1c. Sample MILS, page 3.

(continued)

- If you feel dizzy, sit up slowly, put legs over the side of the bed, and stay there for a few minutes.

- Some people think because Thiazides are taken to remove fluids from the body, they must restrict fluid or water intake. This is wrong. Continue to drink normal amounts of fluid.

- When you first take Thiazide drugs, you may urinate more often. If this is very inconvenient, do NOT stop taking the drug. Call your doctor. Perhaps they can be taken at a different time.

- Thiazide drugs may cause your body to lose salt and water. Your doctor may recommend foods rich in potassium such as bananas or oranges, or you may be given a prescription for a potassium drug. Do not take potassium supplements unless prescribed by your doctor.

- Thiazides may make you more likely to sunburn. Avoid too much heat, sunlight, saunas, or hot baths.

Check yourself:

- If you have shortness of breath or swelling of hands or feet, call your doctor.

Figure 4.1d. Sample MILS, page 4.

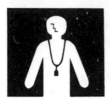

Information your Doctor needs:

Do you have or have you ever had:

- An allergic reaction to thiazides or "sulfa" drugs?
- Diabetes, kidney or liver disease?
- Gout?
- Lupus erythematosus?

Are you taking:

- Heart medicines (Digoxin, Digitalis)?
- Lithium carbonate or phenobarbital?
- Medicines for diabetes?
- Narcotic pain medications?
- Alcohol?

Possible side effects:

These can be bothersome at times. But do not stop taking Thiazides unless your doctor tells you.

Figure 4.1e. Sample MILS, page 5.

(continued)

- You may experience confusion, weakness, or clumsiness especially when standing, when you first take Thiazide drugs. Elderly people may notice these effects more than others.
- You may find that you are allergic to Thiazides and get a rash, hives and an increased sensitivity to sunlight (severe sunburn).
- You may have reduced appetite, indigestion, stomach cramps, diarrhea, vomiting, headaches, or blurred vision.

If these or other side effects bother you, call your doctor.

Call your Doctor:

If you have diarrhea or vomiting.

Please remember:
- If you want more information about this drug, ask you doctor for a more technical leaflet, the professional package insert.
- Tell your doctor *all* medications you are currently taking, whether they are prescription or non-prescription drugs.
- Keep this and all drugs out of reach of children.
- If there is a chance you are or will become pregnant or breast-feed a child, please contact your doctor before taking this drug.
- Keep this leaflet for further reference.

10/82   62M   © 1982 Retired Persons Services, Inc.

Figure 4.1f. Sample MILS, page 6.

There are a number of policy issues we face or have faced in preparing the MILS. One is assurance of accuracy. What steps do we follow to prepare each MILS? First, AARP Pharmacy writes preliminary drafts with initial review and changes by FDA. Second, FDA versions are reviewed and revised by two of our consultants, one a physician and the other a pharmacist, each with expertise in drugs and the elderly. They each rewrite the material and gear it to the elderly. A third consultant, also a physician and geriatrician, critiques each version for medical accuracy and completeness. Then AARP Pharmacy, combining FDA and consultant texts, rewrites each and gears it to the elderly layperson in simple language. Finally, FDA and the reviewing consultant again review each for content and style and to iron out any inconsistencies.

A second issue concerns preparing an MILS when there are questions of marginal efficacy. Just because our members are prescribed a particular medication (ie, a vasodilator), do we simply tell them how to take it and about its common side effects, or do we also have a responsibility to alert them if a medication has received a possibly or probably effective rating? In the cases of nylidrin (Arlidin) and cyclandelate (Cyclospasmol), for example, after talking at length with our consultants, we decided to include a warning on the MILS stating "the National Academy of Sciences, National Research Council, and FDA have classified this drug as 'possibly effective' and recommended it be reevaluated. We suggest you discuss its use with your doctor."

A third issue concerns updates and revisions. When is the appropriate time to revise? How much attention should be given to new reports in the medical literature? What significance should be given to anecdotal evidence? It was agreed that MILS should be revised on an as-needed basis. For example, in the case of cimetidine (Tagamet), we rewrote the MILS when it was documented in the literature that antacids should not be taken concurrently with cimetidine. We removed all the old Tagamet leaflets from our 10 pharmacies. Our consultants agreed there is no need to react to every citation in the literature, but if something is reported that is significant, the MILS are revised.

A fourth issue concerns acceptance of the MILS. We were originally concerned that physicians might react negatively after learning we had provided prescription drug information to their patients. We have received no negative comments about the MILS from physicians, and in fact have been gratified with their reaction. Although our pharmacists reacted negatively initially to the assumed increased workload, they are supportive.

One of the major arguments leveled against mandatory patient package inserts (PPIs) was that these leaflets will scare people — people either won't read them, or if they do, they'll immediately stop taking their medication. We were interested in measuring patient acceptance of the leaflets, and in August 1982 performed an evaluation of the program with FDA to see what, if any, impact the leaflets had. We surveyed by mail 2,400 AARP members who had received one of four prescriptions from us. Seventy percent responded to our survey. The overwhelming majority gave the leaflets a strongly positive rating. Of those indicating they had received the leaflet, 95% said they read it; 76% said they kept it.

The great majority (65%) found the leaflet "very useful" and 29% reported that it was "slightly useful." Only 6% of the respondents said the leaflet was not useful. Most (56%) said they had discussed the leaflet with another person. Although family members were the most common group with whom patients discussed the leaflet, 22% said they had talked about the leaflet with their physician.

Most (69%) said the MILS provided them with information, and many (42%) said the MILS made them feel better about taking their medicine. The leaflets made only a small minority (2%) feel worse. This research is described in more detail in the February 1984 *American Journal of Public Health.*

This preliminary evaluation seems to warrant several conclusions — the MILS program is generally viewed in a positive manner by the elderly who receive the leaflets, and these leaflets *might* result in higher patient acceptance of their medicines, as well as potentially increasing utilization, thereby having a positive health impact.

Recently Smith Kline & French awarded a grant to Dr Jerry Avorn to conduct a second evaluation of our leaflet program. This evaluation will attempt to address such issues as:

• Impact of the MILS on the knowledge of recipients concerning safety and side effects

• Effect of MILS on attitudes about medications

• Effect of MILS on compliance

We expect results by early 1985.

In closing, I would like to suggest some future studies including well designed interventions, randomized and with a control group if possible. The design should consider the expected impact so that the appropriate numbers of patients can be selected. Interventions should be well described so they can be replicated. Finally, it is important that each audience, physician, pharmacist, and patient be examined separately.

Chapter 5

PHYSICIAN INSTRUCTIONS TO THE PATIENT

Kenneth F. Lampe, PhD

Although only 11% of the U.S. population is 65 or older, 30% of prescriptions are written for this population group. Much effort has been expended to identify factors unique to drug use in this population. That particular age-related problems in the use of drugs exist and that elderly patients should receive special consideration when determining the dosage of some drugs are accepted facts. However, realization of the twin goals of safe and effective drug utilization remains unfulfilled despite major educational programs by organizations of physicians, pharmacists, nurses, public health workers, the pharmaceutical industry, government agencies, and associations for the elderly for their members and for the public.

For an individual patient, certain problems may be identified and addressed by the physician. These include the seriousness and prognosis of the disease, its chronicity, and the interaction with other pathophysiology and disease presented by that patient. It is within the physician's function to determine the goal of therapeutic intervention, including whether treatment is even desirable, and to select an appropriate drug and dosage after consideration of all factors that might modify the response to the drug. This much, including adjustments for age-related alterations in pharmacokinetics and pharmacodynamics, applies to any patient population.

Certain problems associated with the actual taking of the drug, some of which are more common in the elderly, require far more physician effort and attention. These problems have been dealt with extensively elsewhere, so only a few will be mentioned here in review.

One of the more prominent problems involves the possibility of drug interactions, which can be enhanced in the elderly for various reasons. Patients can be treated by and receive prescriptions from several physicians at the same time. This can apply even to physicians of the same specialty if the patient perceives the conditions as unrelated. For example, the patient might go to one physician for "heart medicine" and to another who successfully cleared up a friend's ankle edema. The problem is exacerbated by automatic refills and telephone prescribing and by a patient's use of more than one pharmacy. Drug interactions also are related to the exchange of drugs with others and to the failure of the patient, and sometimes the physician, to perceive OTC medications as "drugs."

There also are numerous reasons for poor compliance, especially in this age group. Erratic use can be due to diminished memory or to poor comprehension of a dose schedule. Drugs can be discontinued if the disease is characterized by essentially silent symptoms, as in hypertension, glaucoma, and diabetes. Patients may be self-selective in their medication; the drug for pain in an arthritic joint, for example, may be identified as more important than the diuretic. Drugs that cause unpleasant side effects, even trivial ones, may not be taken. The patient can become discouraged with a chronic illness and feel that medication is useless. He or she may be concerned that the drug might be habit-forming. Financial constraints are a serious problem. It is revealing to observe a patient ask a pharmacist to price the drugs for each prescription so that he or she can determine which ones he or she can afford to have filled. A patient might take only half of the prescribed dose each day to make the costly drug last longer. Overdose errors can result from measurement failures, eagerness to get well, or inappropriate response when the patient realizes that that a dose has been missed.

One of the often-proposed remedies for inappropriate drug utilization is better physician-patient communication. However, it is important to define the necessary elements of that communication. It has been shown (Whartman SA, et al: *Med Care* 1983; 21:886–891) that compliance is not a function of patient *satisfaction* with the patient-physician encounter, but rather with the *quality* of communication. No correlation related to drug compliance could be demonstrated with the patient's perception of his or her interaction with the physician, the duration of the visit, the answers to his or her questions, an apparent appreciation of the patient's anxiety or discomfort, or the thoroughness of the examination.

If a good bedside (or deskside) manner is not the answer, then more attention to the quality of the information may be important in improving the safe and effective utilization of drugs. One approach to strengthening physician-patient communication is to provide the patient with written information concerning the drugs that have been prescribed. Printed information for the patient to take home serves this function, and various organizations, including the American Medical Association, supply such information. These are called Patient Medication Instruction sheets (PMIs). The text and format for the PMIs have been developed in cooperation with the United States Pharmacopeial Convention (USP).

It is expected that the PMIs reduce the risk of improper drug use, decrease the incidence of preventable and serious drug reactions, and improve patient compliance. The information is intended to augment the oral communication between the patient and physician during the office visit. Particular care has been taken to keep the PMIs as simple and as short as possible; to include only commonly accepted, scientific statements about drugs; and to use easily understood language. This prevents an information overload and reduces the risk of providing inconsistent information to the patient.

Each PMI consists of a 5 1/2- by 8 1/2-inch sheet, printed on both sides, with information about a particular drug (for example, erythromycin) or a drug class (for example, the thiazide diuretics). These sheets are supplied at nominal cost in tear-off pads. On the pad backing, the generic and trade names of relevant drugs are given. A space is provided at the top of the PMI for the physician to write in the specific drug prescribed along with the name of the patient and any special instructions concerning the medication. By April 1984, pads will be available for 82 drugs or drug classes. On the basis of NDTI data on outpatient prescriptions, it can be concluded that all of the 200 most commonly prescribed drugs — approximately 90% of all prescribed oral medications — are represented.

Each PMI begins with an introductory statement, "This sheet tells you about the medicine your doctor has prescribed for you. If any of this information causes you special concern, check with your doctor." This addresses the problem that has been raised by some physicians, and for which we have inadequate data, that drug information may actually decrease trust in the doctor's judgment and result in diminished compliance. For some patients, this may be the case. A certain percentage of patients are not interested. There is an apparent desire for additional information by many, however, as evidenced by a recent study that found that 17 million American homes possessed a copy of the *Physician's Desk Reference* (PDR).

The PMI makes a brief, simple statement about the purpose of the medication, for example, "It is used to treat high blood pressure." All have the admonition, "Take this medicine only as directed by your doctor." The patient is then instructed, "Before using this medicine, be sure to tell your doctor if you. . . ." If there are any particularly important potential drug interactions or pathophysiologic states that would be of concern with a particular drug, they are included here. Otherwise, there is a set of circumstances that most commonly includes, "are allergic to any medicine, are pregnant or intend to become pregnant while using this medicine, are breast-feeding, are taking any other prescription or nonprescription medication, or have any other medical problems."

The "proper use of this medicine" section is particularly aimed at compliance. The first element is dosage, which may be concerned with patient-selected modifications in quantity or with continued application. An example of the latter might be, "If blood pressure is not treated, it can cause serious problems, such as heart failure, blood vessel disease, stroke, or kidney disease. This drug will not cure your blood pressure, but it does help to control it. Therefore, you must continue to take it — even if you feel well — if you expect to keep your blood pressure down." The second segment of this section begins, "If you miss a dose of this medicine. . . ." The appropriate response is inserted.

There is a brief section on "precautions while using this medicine." Included are such matters as first-dose effects, precautions about driving, mention of OTC products that should be avoided, and, in some instances, instructions on what the patient can do to relieve or minimize predictable side effects, such as orthostatic hypotension.

A listing of side effects appears, but PMIs do not present a "laundry list" of all reported adverse reactions. Those selected are divided into two labeled groups, "side effects that should be reported to your doctor" and "side effects that might not require medical attention." The second group includes a statement, "These possible side effects may go away during treatment; however, if they persist, contact your doctor." Because side effects concerning impotence are so subject to psychological induction, they have been deliberately omitted.

The PMIs close with a statement in fine print, "The information in this PMI is selective and does not cover all the possible uses, actions, precautions, side effects, or interactions with this medicine." The inclusion of this statement is to emphasize to the physician that the PMI is not a substitute for the explanations and instructions on drugs that should be given to the patient and it is *not* intended as a legal instrument of informed consent.

We feel that the use of the PMIs can help reduce the cost of care by decreasing unnecessary visits or calls to the physician. They might also help to improve patient satisfaction with visits and with the physician-patient relationship. For those elderly patients for whom it is necessary that a spouse, child, or sitter manage the administration of the medication (who were not in direct communication with the physician) the written instruction should prove invaluable in improving the safe use of the drug. It would be an interesting research project to compare compliance and knowledge of the prescribed drug between a PMI- and a non-PMI-supplied patient population.

As evidenced by use and by reorders of PMIs from prescribing physicians, the response has been encouraging. However, we do not feel that these instruction sheets are being used in adequate numbers. A survey made during the early part of the PMI program examined the reasons for nonuse. A single factor was dominant: Some physicians were opposed to patient information in general and to the use of PMIs in particular. This could be correlated to the age of the physician, the older physician being less sympathetic to the need for patient education. Because the American Medical Association is committed to the Patient Medication Information program as an important approach to improve the safe and effective use of drugs, ways are being sought to convince these physicians of its importance. Currently, the AMA is preparing a Spanish language version of the PMIs. This should be of particular value in the elderly Spanish immigrant with fragmentary knowledge of English, especially if he or she has a non-Spanish-speaking physician.

The AMA would appreciate any suggestions that might increase the impact of this program on quality medical care for all patients (and especially the elderly, for whom, as was noted, a large percentage of drug prescriptions are written).

Chapter 6

SELF-MEDICATION WITH OVER-THE-COUNTER DRUGS

Albert G. Eckian, MD

Self-medication is the most prevalent form of medical care among the elderly, as it is among all Americans. Moreover, there are extraordinary demographic and sociological forces at work that will cause a dynamic growth of self-medication in the elderly over the next 40 years. The demographic changes are embodied in what is commonly called the "graying of America." The sociological shifts are reflected in our rapidly changing health care delivery systems.

Let us briefly examine the major demographic shifts. The current elderly population — those 65 and over — constitutes approximately 12% of our total U.S. population. In 40 years, those 65 and over will be approximately 23% of our population. Although the percentage gains are impressive, the absolute numbers are staggering. The 65 plus age group is 28 million strong in 1984. In 40 years, this group will more than double in number to over 58 million. It is therefore an unavoidable conclusion that there will be a much greater need for all sorts of medical services and products by the rapidly growing elderly population as each year goes by. We can expect to see more self-medication, more home nursing visits, more hospice visits, more specialized dietary programs, and so on, even if current per capita utilization remains unchanged.

Now let us look at the dramatic sociological changes that are occurring in our health care delivery system. The traditional providers — mainly the private physician and hospital — are now complemented by other providers who have developed or will soon attain a national reach. The visiting nurse, hospice, home renal dialysis, independent dietician, health maintenance organization, freestanding satellite clinic, the nurse practitioner, home hyperalimentation, and at-home chemotherapy are but a few examples of additional providers or services that have grown dramatically over the past 20 years.

Here are just a few figures that demonstrate the changing patterns of health care. In 1978 the State of Florida had 75 patients on home renal dialysis. In 1982, there were over 300 patients on home renal dialysis. That is an increase of 400% in just 4 years. What about hospice? In 1978 there were 59 hospice programs in the entire country. In 1982 — just 4 years later — there were nearly 1,000 hospice programs. That is a 1700% increase. What about the Visiting Nurse Associations? In 1961 the Visiting Nurse Association of New York City made 294,000 visits. In 1981 they made over 1 million visits.

In tandem with the decentralization of health care, today's consumer has aggressively embraced a wellness-driven mode of health care that includes more healthful eating habits, exercise programs, stress alleviation and preventive medical care. An ever-growing number of Americans are taking a hands-on approach to their medical care — learning through books, pamphlets, television, and hospital-based health education programs. There has been a proliferation of home medical devices, home diagnostics, and in-home services to complement an already established system of self-medication.

Now just where does self-medication fit into the health care delivery of the elderly? A recently completed consumer survey assessed the health care practices of the U.S. population with respect to the generally minor and self-limiting conditions that are traditionally associated with self-medication. Adults over the age of 65 reported an average of 4.2 health problems during a two-week period. Of these health problems, 35% were treated with non-prescription medicines. Older consumers using nonprescription medicines reported successful and safe use of these products. When asked why their nonprescription medicines had been discontinued, 87% reported that the medical problem had "gone away". Only 6% of the elderly reported that the non-prescription medicine had failed to work. Two percent stated that they had run out of medicine, and another 2% reported that their physicians advised a change or discontinuation of the medication. Less than 1% reported an unfavorable reaction to the nonprescription medications used.

In the same survey, 92% of the older individuals expressed satisfaction with the product they had used; and 91% indicated that they would use the same type of nonprescription medicine again if the health problem recurred.

The survey has also dispelled some widespread beliefs regarding the health care practices of older people. We commonly hear that the elderly population is hooked on medication. Some would have us believe that they are popping pills constantly. We are also told that the elderly are overly dependent on physicians. We looked at these beliefs with respect to the generally minor and self-limiting conditions that are traditionally associated with self-medication. What we found was that 35% of the health problems were not treated at all. The consumer would just tolerate the condition. Furthermore, about 11% of the conditions were treated primarily with a home remedy. Therefore, almost half of the health care problems didn't even enter the traditional systems of health care delivery.

When elderly consumers did use nonprescription medications, they reported that treatment was usually for only a day or two and was also usually limited to one medication. Therefore, with respect to nonprescription medications, our elderly population is not hooked on them. They are not popping pills indiscriminately. On the contrary, they are extraordinarily judicious with respect to OTC medications.

Regarding physician consultations, 14% of the elderly consult a physician for the generally minor, self-limiting conditions included in our study. This 14% figure reflects an appropriately higher level of concern for overall health by the elderly patient when compared to the general population (all ages), who consult a physician for 9% of these health problems.

In summary, self-medication with nonprescription medications is the dominant mode of health care delivery among the elderly. The medications are used safely and with good effect. Additionally, it is widely acknowledged that nonprescription medicines provide one of the most cost-efficient ways of treating acute illnesses and maintaining wellness in terms of both time and money. Nothing short of true prevention — such as immunizations, exercise, and good eating habits — is more cost-efficient.

There can be nothing but optimism about the growing role of self-medication in the elderly population group. The powerful demographic and sociological forces mentioned will move into the hands of the elderly consumer much more responsibility for his or her own health care. And that is where the responsibility belongs.

HEALTH EDUCATION AND INFORMATION: THE FOUNDATION OF SELF-MEDICATION

The foundation of increased self-medication among the elderly is health information and education. Pharmaceutical manufacturers participate in the dissemination of information, but their efforts are only part of vigorous activity in many other areas. Hospitals now actively promote health education programs in areas such as arthritis, diabetes, heart disease, and hypertension. Physicians are incorporating more preventive medicine into their practices. Foundations disseminate information on virtually every disease. Hundreds of health care books, magazines, pamphlets, and audiotapes are now readily available. Health care is very popular on television, radio, and in newspaper columns. The outreach of visiting nurses, the hospice, and similar programs is based on individual patient education.

The consumer's assimilation of health care knowledge sets the stage for effective self-medication. The manufacturers focus their efforts on the three pillars of self-medication. First is the development of a drug ingredient that is intrinsically safe. It is known that medications are not absolutely safe for all people. However, it is also known that there are a large number of drug ingredients wherein there is a wide margin between the therapeutic dose and the toxic dose. This margin of safety provides a buffer zone for the occasional but inevitable misadventure that will occur in self-medication. Misadventures occur with all drugs, both prescription and nonprescription, but those that are nonprescription must have this built-in safety margin.

The second pillar to self-medication in the elderly is the preparation of label copy that is understandable. Generally, comprehensible label copy is not a major barrier. Utilizing simple language and diagrams one can devise adequate directions for use, including cautions and warnings.

Finally, to self-medicate effectively, one must be able to make an accurate assessment of the symptom or illness that is at hand. Traditionally, self-medication has been used to alleviate the acute symptoms of self-limiting ailments such as the common cold, a headache, heartburn, or episodic constipation. However, chronic conditions have also been treated via self-medication, including the use of aspirin for arthritis, insulin for diabetes, or topical selenium sulfide for dandruff. Prevention is also well established in self-medication — witness the daily use of fluorides to prevent dental caries.

As our informed elderly become more knowledgeable, we should expect more chronic conditions and preventive modes to be handled through self-medication. The condition assessment and the design of the health care plan may occur more frequently in conjunction with the patient's physician. However, after a proper assessment has been made, access to safe, effective, well-labeled OTCs should be encouraged. The extent of professional supervision for a chronic condition — if needed at all — can be designed on an individual basis. For example, the management of arthritis with aspirin is now commonplace, as is the use of antacids for ulcer disease. The professional diagnosis of these illnesses and the establishment of a professional care plan should not preclude direct access to the appropriate medications via over-the-counter sale. There are many more chronic conditions wherein patients could participate more actively in the care plan if more medications were available over-the-counter. Even now, many physicians establish care plans that are based upon the long-term, intelligent self-administration of prescription medications. The patient will receive PRN refills for his or her medication with only occasional checkups — perhaps every 6 months to 1 year — if there are no complicating factors. This type of care plan represents a transitional phenomenon that acknowledges the informed patient's ability to take a more active role in managing chronic conditions. Hypertension, diabetes, ulcer disease, heart disease, and arthritis are all good examples of conditions wherein physicians are turning over more management to the patient. The foundation of this transformation has been patient education. The advent of more nonprescription medications to treat chronic conditions will be an appropriate outgrowth of the extraordinary medical and health education progress that has been made by the consumer over the past several years.

Rx TO OTC DRUG SWITCHES

Where will all these new OTC drugs for chronic conditions come from? The answer, quite simply, is from our own backyard. There has been an extraordinary amount of interest lately in Rx to OTC drug switches. The ability to transfer a drug from prescription (Rx) to OTC status is not new. The law clearly states that if a drug can be sold over-the-counter then it must be sold over-the-counter. Over the past 40 years pharmaceutical companies have generally preferred prescription-only status for their new products. Generally, OTC sale has not been sought. However, the advent of the OTC drug review has changed our perceptions and our behavior.

The 17 OTC Advisory Review Panels have examined virtually all OTC drug ingredients, making 37 recommendations for Rx to OTC drug switches in the process. Some of the advisory panel recommendations have involved bringing to the OTC market ingredients that were formerly limited to prescription-only sale. Other switches have involved increasing OTC ingredient dosages to the same level as found in prescription drugs. The FDA has agreed with a substantial number of the proposed switches. Indeed, FDA has recently proposed the switch of a few ingredients on their own.

In view of the new environment surrounding health care delivery, pharmaceutical companies have gone to a great deal of effort to explore the general parameters surrounding the Rx to OTC switch phenomenon. Industry has utilized its own personnel, trade associations, and highly regarded technical consultants from all around the country to explore the science, the economics, the regulatory mechanisms, and the public policy ramifications of switches. Several companies have also submitted applications to FDA to switch prescription drugs to nonprescription status. Many of these petitions have received favorable FDA review. Most readers of this book are familiar with some of these recently switched products such as the triprolidine HCl-pseudoephedrine HCl combination (Actifed®), the dexbrompheniramine maleate-pseudoephedrine sulfate combination (Drixoral® , oxymetazoline HCl (Afrin®), and diphenhydramine HCl (Benylin®).

I think we are on the threshold of a whole new generation of safe and effective OTC medications. There are a large number of drugs that physicians have prescribed for years — often decades — that are now well understood, very safe, and are good candidates for OTC status. Informed consumers have the medical and health knowledge to readily integrate new frontiers of self-medication into their health care programs. It is in the consumer's interest for us to support the Rx to OTC switch. Some would say that more nonprescription drugs are a basic legal right. The economic justification is self-evident. With the nation's health care bill now well in excess of $300 billion annually, we must provide the elderly consumer with greater access to health care tools at a lower total cost.

In discussing the Rx to OTC switch, we must keep in mind the three pillars of self-medication mentioned earlier. The ingredients must have a high margin of safety; there must be understandable labeling; and there must be a method of illness assessment — be it self-diagnosis or professional diagnosis. Most importantly, we are not talking about switching highly toxic drugs, such as oral digoxin, that have a very small safety margin. Nor are we talking about switching drugs for which understandable labeling — for whatever reason — cannot be written. However, even with these precautions, virtually all of us could go through our PDR®s item by item and come up with several more pharmaceuticals that are suitable for self-medication — and therefore are serious candidates for switch evaluation by the FDA.

THE PERCEPTION OF THE ELDERLY

Let us pause now to examine some other common perceptions and misconceptions about the elderly. Traditionally, the elderly have been viewed as poor, sick, disabled, and enfeebled — just putting in their time until inevitable death. This perception of the elderly still lingers today. However, if we talk to the elderly themselves, their viewpoint is quite different. The elderly generally consider themselves to be in good health, despite chronic conditions. In the survey noted earlier, 94% of those 65 and older considered their health to be "average" or better. Sixty-five percent of the elderly assessed their health as "fairly good" or "excellent." Also, the elderly are mobile — although not as mobile as a 30- or 40-year-old. Only 5% of the elderly require institutional care; 95% are out in the mainstream of life. The fact is that the elderly population is alive and well, vigorous and energetic, and growing daily in number. These individuals are well informed, well educated, and generally knowledgeable.

Admittedly, in today's elderly population there are still a significant number of people who were brought up in the tradition of medical dependency. Basically, this consumer knew little about health care and relied totally upon his or her personal physician. However, even now, that is all changing very rapidly. Today, the elderly ranks are full of patients who appropriately question each procedure, test, or medication; who seek second opinions; and who play a big role in the health care decision-making process. This is the informed consumer who is ready for Rx to OTC drug switches. Huge savings would result if physicians and hospitals would aggressively provide the elderly with more opportunities for the self-management of common chronic ailments such as arthritis, heart disease, diabetes, gout, asthma, bronchitis, and so on. We need no new technology — it abounds all around us. We do not need new medicines — there are plenty of therapeutic agents. What we need is more information, more education, and then increased access to the appropriate health care tools be they medications, home diagnostics, or home medical devices.

SPECIAL LABELING FOR THE ELDERLY

One of the most important topics for today is the question of special labeling for the elderly. In order to address the specific needs of a specific population group, one must have scientific knowledge. In the case of the elderly, there is some knowledge regarding biological systems. We know, for example, that gastrointestinal transit time usually increases with age. Glomerular filtration rate generally decreases with age. The fat to lean body mass ratio usually increases with age. Hepatic metabolism probably decreases for some enzyme systems. What we don't know, however, is how these and the many other biological changes that occur with age affect the total absorption, distribution, pharmacokinetic profile, and therapeutic activity of specific drug ingredients in finite age groups. Therefore, scientifically sound labeling based *solely upon chronological age* is currently not feasible for most drug ingredients.

A much more useful and scientific approach is that adopted by the OTC Advisory Review Panels. These panels identified *specific medical conditions* for which ingredient labeling was appropriate. Many of the medical conditions identified by OTC review panels are much more common in older age groups and thereby address the needs of the elderly. For example, if a given ingredient is to be used with caution in people with heart disease, hypertension, or prostatism, we have, by the intrinsic nature of these medical conditions, cautions that serve mainly older age groups. Our current medical knowledge supports condition-specific labeling not only for indications but also for cautions and warnings.

A brief look at the problems associated with chronologic age-specific labeling indicates that this type of labeling will probably be appropriate in only very limited circumstances. The aging process is extraordinarily complex. Gerontologists generally agree that the changes in biological functions that characterize aging probably start in the 30s, if not earlier. The changes proceed at different rates, depending upon an individual's genetics and total environment. By the age of 40, 50, or 60 the accumulated changes in physiologic functioning become clearly visible and we are perceptibly "older."

The pivotal distinction that must be made is between chronological age and physiological age. We all know people in their seventies who have all the apparent vigor of other individuals 10 or 20 years younger. Conversely, a person of 55 might well have physiological changes equivalent to the "average" 70-year-old. We cannot, therefore, increase or decrease an elderly person's medication dosage just because of chronological age. Indeed, many have suggested that the amount of variability *within* specific older age groups might far exceed the average variability *between* age groups. The variabilities of pharmacological parameters both within and between age groups have not been well demonstrated for most drug ingredients. Therefore, at least for the time being, condition-specific labeling should be relied upon as the most accurate and most scientifically sound form of labeling when considering the needs of the elderly.

Future clinical testing may delineate age-specific changes in a drug's metabolism that will warrant special product labeling. The FDA, of course, would have to establish appropriate criteria for such clinical trials. Also, it would probably not be productive to retest nonprescription drugs that have wide margins of safety and that generally present few problems for elderly patients. Perhaps any future age-specific testing should be limited to those drugs where the therapeutic and toxic doses converge.

Given that condition-specific labeling will accommodate the needs of the elderly for the vast majority of nonprescription ingredients, we should now focus on a current challenge to FDA and to the industry. Nonprescription medications are labeled with abundant amounts of information. There is the name of the active ingredient, the dosage strength, indications, directions for use, as well as cautions, warnings, and drug interactions. We can anticipate that as the OTC drug review continues we will get more — not less — labeling information. The big challenge is not finding information; there is plenty of information for OTC product labels. What we need are alternative ways to present and display that information in more readable and more digestible formats. As the amount of information required on OTC labels continues to explode, the label sizes stay the same. Indeed, packaging laws require that manufacturers not deceive their consumers by putting small amounts of medicine in extraordinarily large packages. Therefore, we can anticipate alternative approaches to labeling and packaging that will respond to the ever-increasing amounts of useful and required medication information.

We do not know today the best way to meet the labeling and packaging challenges. However, in the next few years labeling and packaging alternatives can be developed if there is a concerted effort by all.

In summary, the outlook for self-medication by the elderly is bright. We have an expanding base of medically knowledgeable consumers who want more control over their individual health care programs. We have skyrocketing medical costs stimulating public policies that demand cost-efficiency. We have a receptive regulatory environment and appropriate regulatory mechanisms to provide for more nonprescription medicines via the judicious switch of selected prescription-only pharmaceuticals to nonprescription status. We have a high level of awareness of the aging process, and the outlook is for condition-specific labeling that addresses the changes in health status that occur in the elderly. We have an abundance of labeling information (and more coming) that will stimulate alternative labeling and packaging formats. All indicators point to self-medication as a continuing mainstay in a changing health care delivery system. The contributions we all make from our respective professional disciplines will be extremely important, benefiting not only the elderly but individuals of all ages.

PART 3

A GLOBAL PROGRAM OF HEALTH CARE FOR THE ELDERLY

Chapter 7

THE WORLD HEALTH ORGANIZATION'S GLOBAL PROGRAM OF HEALTH CARE FOR THE ELDERLY

M.N. Graham Dukes, MD

Whenever the name of the World Health Organization (WHO) is mentioned in a developed, industrialized country, a certain number of the people present will be found to be living with the conviction that the organization works only in developing countries. That impression isn't surprising; a global organization is bound to make its greatest efforts where there is the greatest need, and quite obviously this means that proportionately more of WHO's resources must be devoted to the very pressing problems of health in the third world. Very often these countries can benefit from the technical knowledge and experience of industrialized countries, whether it be in pumping up fresh water in the desert or conquering tropical disease.

There are fields, however, where almost the reverse applies. If one looks at the fate that awaits the elderly in many industrialized societies, one may well find that it is far less pleasant than that in more traditional societies. The way in which religious orders care for old people in one developing country or the way in which they play an integrated role in family life as long as people live in many others are things that many Western countries can learn from.

The question of drugs and the elderly is, by contrast, a universal one, although it shows nuances as one goes across the world. The problem has many different facets, but let me concentrate on one of them, namely, the dissemination and use of existing knowledge. This is a problem with which the World Health Organization is all too familiar. Three-quarters of our health problems — perhaps more — are due not to the fact that mankind does not know enough, but because we do not use the knowledge we already have. One does not have to look very long at this field before seeing what is wrong. There are some vast discrepancies between what is known about the kinetics, the value, and the risks of many drugs in the elderly and the prescribing patterns one finds in practice. That sounds at once like a grave rebuke to the practitioner. I am not sure that it is. The fault lies much deeper, in our whole way of putting facts to work. A lot of the knowledge about the particular characteristics of old age and the way drugs act in that period of life has only emerged during the last generation, and particularly during the last decade, in other words, after doctors now in practice received their training or at least entered medical school. Medical school curricula still do not always devote as much time to this question as one would like, in spite of the high proportion of the elderly in the population. Postgraduate education is there, but not everywhere, and on such matters it often reaches only a fraction of practitioners, often the fraction that is in any case most conscientious and best-informed. The challenge is very largely a question of how we get the essential facts on this matter across to the prescriber so that he or she will not merely remember them but also put them to work.

How does WHO tackle a problem like this? We think we have found the seed to a solution working in four stages.

The first stage was to come to a reasonable consensus on the general facts. This we succeeded in doing, reaching a broader measure of agreement than we ever dared to expect, in a Technical Group meeting held at Thonex, Switzerland, in 1980. The group, whose report was published in the journal *Drugs* a year later, studied the whole demographic background and looked at existing prescribing patterns and their consequences to identify the real practical problems. It went on to look at a host of other matters and to set out general principles — on kinetics, compliance, the need for drug treatment, problems of adverse reactions, labeling, and many more.

With this basis laid, the second stage was tackled by holding a meeting, this time largely European, to hammer out some of the more technical aspects, at Schlangenbad, West Germany, later in 1980. Looking this time at the way drug regulatory authorities and clinical pharmacologists might help to put matters straight, we again reached a remarkable consensus, without any resort to vague compromises. We looked at matters as concrete as regulatory standards, estrogen therapy for osteoporosis, and the astonishing variation in the range of so-called geriatric drugs on sale from one country to the next, and yet we agreed.

We could now come to grips with the third stage. Two years ago, the WHO program on the Health of the Elderly set up a working group of highly experienced geriatricians and kineticists to produce a handbook on drugs and the elderly for the prescriber. The handbook was written in record time, and in August 1983, it was thoroughly checked by a global group of experts at a meeting held in Iceland. It is now finished and publication is anticipated during the summer of 1984. Building as it does on the consensus of the earlier meetings, it gives the prescriber down-to-earth, practical advice. It summarizes the practical principles and pitfalls and goes on to deal in short monographs with almost all those groups of drugs and individual drugs that are or should be used in the elderly — dosage, indications, risks, and all.

We know very well that there are books on this theme already, but we also know what a very small percentage of the world's physician population ever gets around to reading them. Naturally, there can and must be some adaptation of the text to deal with purely regional or national needs, but we must ensure that we are working with national bodies, such as medical associations, to produce adapted texts. What emerges, we feel sure, will be a global network of small books, available at very low cost, slipping readily into the doctor's pocket and going as well to medical students and a range of medical auxiliaries. There also seems to be a place for an equivalent popular volume, in part for old people themselves and in part for those who are caring for them, including their families.

At the World Health Organization we do hope, and we very much believe, that in this we shall be making a real advance, supported by the organizations working with us, to make drug treatment in the elderly better and safer, wherever in the world it is used.

PART 4

AGENDA FOR GERIATRIC DRUG RESEARCH

Chapter 8

SETTING THE AGENDA
FOR GERIATRIC DRUG RESEARCH

T. Franklin Williams, MD

Part of the difficulty in setting the agenda for geriatric drug research is that much has already been said and many have called for more investigation. Another difficulty is that we are in such an early stage of addressing specific issues about the relationship of drugs to older people that much work still needs to be done. Furthermore, the commitment to research on drugs related to the elderly is still very small compared to the rapidly expanding number of older people, who are inevitably going to be using a sizeable number of drugs. Partially this is because investigators have not brought forward challenging research proposals, and partially it is due to the competition for the research dollar. Also, after talking to persons from the pharmaceutical industry, I have learned that there has been very little direct addressing of issues related to aging and drug effects. Looking at all these factors, I think we have a stake in trying to expand our commitment in this field. If there is any message, it is that we all have much farther to go to address research issues on drug use and older people. I will try to highlight a few of the areas that should be on our agenda.

DIFFERENTIATION OF AGING FROM DISEASE

First of all, as a basic starting point, we still need to learn much more about aging per se and how to differentiate aging from disease. What changes in the normal — biological or psychological — state are brought by the passage of time? Then, can we in turn relate those changes to responses to drugs? The importance of understanding age-related changes cannot be overestimated because the more we learn the more we find that most declines in bodily function that occur in the later years are due to disease and not to aging. I want to cite two examples of such new information. One recent study just completed by scientists at the National Institute on Aging's Gerontology Research

Center in Baltimore in collaboration with scientists at The Johns Hopkins Hospital shows that in people in their 70s who had no evidence of even occult coronary artery disease, their maximum cardiac output, under standard stress tests, was as good as that of 25-year-olds.[1] There was no decrement in cardiac output provided they were free of coronary artery disease as established by screening with radioactive thallium scanning to detect even slight degrees of coronary artery disease. About half of the people in their 70s showed no evidence of coronary artery disease even with this advanced type of screening. So we have to rethink our views about an age-related loss in cardiac function, as it appears that the decline so often seen is attributable to disease.

Mental functioning is another area where it has long been assumed that declines occur with age. Recent research has clearly shown that in normal people there is essentially no decline in mental functioning compared to that individuals's own intellectual status earlier in life. This was true of about 80% or more of the people followed in several careful longitudinal studies.[2] There are some slight differences in tests of elements in mental functioning between young and old but overall performance held up extremely well, and that is quite contrary to what has been the general perception of most of our society. Remember that we used to think that everybody eventually became senile; that idea has now been disproven. Today we recognize that a significant number of people suffer from Alzheimer's disease or other dementing disorders but that it is far from a universal affliction. However, most people are still carrying around the lurking suspicion that all of us will lose some mental capacities as we get older even if we don't get a true dementing disorder. The fact is that this is not necessarily true. I think that as we examine brain function with more and more refined techniques we are going to find that aging alone produces minimal changes in the brain and organ functions. That does not mean that there will be no changes in the structural characteristics of body tissues with the passage of time, even without damage from disease or injury. There are changes in connective tissue, changes in the cell membranes, and changes in the nature and extent of the receptor cells for hormones or drugs. We need more research on such changes. But first we need to start from the premise that it is essential to understand and separate out what is aging and what is disease.

A second basic premise is that, in considering the effects of drugs in older people, we have to recognize that most older people do have some chronic disease. Eighty percent or more of people over the age of 65 have at least one diagnosed chronic disease, including such common problems as hearing or visual impairments, arthritis, diabetes, and cardiovascular disease. By the time people reach their 80s, virtually all have at least one diagnosable chronic disease and most have more than one. When we discuss drugs in older people, we must take such facts into account. Consequently we need to study drugs in older people and in the known presence of multiple complex problems. Standard procedure has been to study drug response in a situation free of any compounding variables and this is simply not useful in studying the effects of drugs in older people. The effect and effectiveness of any drug in old people is going to have to be tested and interpreted in the light of a variety of potentially compounding diseases and problems. This issue will be more important as our population over the age of 85 doubles between now and the year 2000.

SPECIFIC BODY CHANGES IN RESPONSE TO DRUGS

Another area that needs consideration and further research is pharmacodynamics. We know very little about aging and changes in drug receptor responses or about what happens inside cells after the drug receptor reaction occurs. At the Gerontology Research Center in Baltimore, current studies are indicating that the regeneration of beta-adrenergic receptors is much slower in older animals compared to younger animals. We need to learn much more about this and, at least in theory, its relation to every type of drug that is commonly used with older people. It has been pointed out that, in the development of drug research, manufacturers usually concentrate on one of a family of potential chemical compounds that seems overall to have the best beneficial to adverse effect ratio for a given purpose. This is, however, usually determined in younger animals or younger people, and it might well be that some other member of a family of compounds would be much more appropriate in older people perhaps because, for example, it has less duration of effect on receptors. Thus there is a whole realm of drug cell interactions to consider in differentiating between old and young members of a species.

I want to caution here that much of the research aimed at identifying changes with aging both in animals and in people compares very young animals or people, adolescents, if you will, with old animals or people. For example, 3- to 6-month-old adolescent rats have been compared with rats aged 24 to 36 months. It appears to be inappropriate to compare such very young, still-maturing animals with very old animals, without including animals in early maturity, say 12 to 15 months of age.

The same problem occurs in humans, for example in studies of drug effects in relation to age when the comparison is of 25-year-olds with 75-year-olds. In such cases, decrements will be found and often classed as age-related effects. In fact, in some instances where this has been explored further it has been found that the apparent decrements in response occurred in early middle adult life. The big differences are seen between, say, 25- and 40-year-olds, with little change beyond that age in humans. This is an important distinction. Some effects have a linear decrement of age beyond the point of maturity, but a number of conclusions from studies have been misleading in attributing to senescence a decrement that really occurs relatively early in life. Probably the correct interpretation would be that there was a more active change during adolescence or early maturity that was actually a biologically normal part of the maturing process, but then a lower level of function becomes appropriate for the stable mature phase of that particular species. Therefore, what we labeled "senescent" wasn't actually an effect of senescence at all. This raises a methodological principle that has to be considered when talking about senescent effects in drug use or about any other physiological studies.

COMPLIANCE

There are other areas that fall outside the biological and basic pharmacological realm but are equally important in research on aging. One of them has to do with the whole question of compliance. I learned years ago in my own research how relatively poor compliance was among people with diabetes. They failed to carry out not only the proper use of drugs but also recommendations for diet, exercise, and urine testing — all the active measures a person with diabetes can take to maintain best health. In one way or another over 60% to 70% had some difficulty with compliance.[3,4] An interesting sidelight was that taking insulin was the only area where compliance was very high, even though 20% to 30% errors in dosage occurred. It seems that the actual fact of giving oneself an injection each day seemed to be enough of an event that almost all diabetics gave themselves their injections. Their compliance in taking oral antidiabetic drugs was no better than in the results of other studies of tablet taking. About 25% failed to take their antidiabetic drug at one time or another. Conceptual models are being developed and tested for their value in guiding efforts to improve compliance. Marshall Becker and colleagues, in their recent review, presented a health decision model in which the recommended elements for study were presented as well as an approach for achieving better compliance.[5] We need to develop individualized strategies in relation to the way a given person responds. I might just illustrate this again from diabetic studies where we found that patients who wanted to be told exactly what to do — about 20% of all diabetics — and who had a doctor who felt that rigid control was the proper method did very well. If such patients had a doctor who had a lackadaisical attitude about diabetes, they did not do very well. And, the reverse was true: if the doctor had a rigid view about diabetes management and the patient a lackadaisical view, again the patient did not do very well. If both doctor and patient had a more relaxed attitude about management of diabetes, then the patient did better than when there was a conflict in approach. In other words, congruence between patient and physician in approach to diabetic management was a distinct advantage. This suggests that we need to be able to define such patient and physician characteristics and adjust our management approaches accordingly.

ADMINISTRATION OF MEDICATIONS
TO THE ELDERLY

We need to have more imaginative efforts to make medication administration as foolproof as possible. Some older people do suffer from forgetfulness and some have physical limitations, and special efforts to develop ways to assist such persons in taking medications would surely be of wide benefit. Consider the question of more use of the transdermal approach for administering medication. Then one can tell by looking at a patch on the arm that the patient has applied the drug and not have to think about whether the pills have or haven't been taken. We need to consider, from a pharmaceutical point of view, ways to package drugs that will minimize confusion for patients. Perhaps a highly individualized approach could be taken where a pharmacist would provide a patient with morning pills in one sealed package, and afternoon pills in another sealed package. Patients or families often have to produce such packages themselves, but I don't see why a pharmacist couldn't do such packaging. At times I have asked a pharmacist to prepare a mixture of insulin because the patient was not capable of mixing it, and that has served the patients very well. Pharmacists can help a lot of people to achieve more effective regimens. This is product development, perhaps, rather than research, but it is an area that needs attention.

There are obviously many areas in which we need much more basic drug research and development. For example, Alzheimer's disease presents a cardinal area in geriatrics where our chance to manage that disease more effectively is going to depend either on discovering a cause that we can prevent or on discovering a medication that will reduce symptoms. Alzheimer's disease presents a vast challenge for research related to aging.

Training

Finally, I want to mention the whole area of training. One of the major missions of the National Institute on Aging is to provide support for training and research and teaching in the fields of aging including use of drugs with older patients. We desperately need more people in our medical and other health profession schools to take the lead in teaching and in research in pharmacological and pharmaceutical issues in aging. The National Institute on Aging will encourage and support additional development of training in this field. The recent *Report on Training in Geriatrics and Gerontology,* prepared by the Public Health Service at the request of Congress, gives a detailed analysis of the needs for more trained professionals in these fields, and makes recommendations for meeting these needs.

REFERENCES

1. Rodenheffer RJ, Gerstenblith G, Becker LC, Fleg JL, Weisfeldt ML, Lakatta EG: Exercise cardiac output is maintained with advancing age in healthy human subjects: Cardiac dilatation and increased stroke volume compensate for a diminished heart rate. *Circulation* 1984; 69(2): 203–213.

2. Schaie KW (ed): *Longitudinal Studies of Adult Psychological Development.* New York, The Guilford Press, 1983.

3. Williams TF, Martin DA, Hogan MD, Watkins JD, Ellis EV, Coyle VC, Lyle IK, Whittinghill M: The clinical picture of diabetic control, studied in four settings. *Amer J Pub Health* 1967; 57:441.

4. Watkins JD, Williams TF, Martin DA, Hogan MD, Anderson E, Coyle V, Cook BA, Lyle IK, McLamb JT: A study of diabetic patients at home. *Amer J Pub Health* 1967; 57:452.

5. Eraka SA, Kirscht JT, Becker MH: Understanding and improving patient compliance. *Annals of Int Med* 1984; 100:258–268.

PART 5

POSTMARKETING SURVEILLANCE AND DRUG UTILIZATION STUDIES IN THE ELDERLY

Chapter 9

DRUG UTILIZATION IN THE GERIATRIC AGE GROUP

Carlene Baum, PhD,
Dianne L. Kennedy, RPh, MPH,
and Mary B. Forbes, RPh

This chapter presents national estimates of age differences in outpatient use of major drug categories. To allow identification of the changes in drug use that accompany increasing age, data cover the entire age spectrum rather than focusing only on the 65 and older age group often defined as the geriatric population. All estimates are based on 1982 data.

METHODS

Data were derived from two subscription data bases purchased by the FDA from IMS America, Ltd. The National Prescription Audit (NPA) is based on a panel of approximately 1,200 computerized pharmacies and provides national estimates of the number of prescriptions dispensed from retail pharmacies. It does not include prescriptions dispensed from other outlets such as supermarkets, discount houses, or mail-order pharmacies. The National Disease and Therapeutic Index (NDTI) is based on a panel of approximately 2,000 private office-based physicians who report on every contact they have with a patient during a specified two-day period.

Drugs recorded during a physician-patient contact can reach the patient through several different channels, as indicated in Table 9.1. Data for this study were limited to drugs that were issued by prescription (ie, "prescription" and "sample and Rx" in Table 9.1). Although the data sets are com-

---

The opinions expressed in this chapter are those of the authors and not necessarily those of the FDA. The authors assume responsibility for the accurate transcription of all data and the mathematical calculations performed by the Drug Use Analysis Branch.

parable for all age groups, the percentage of total NDTI drug issuance by prescription decreases with increasing age. Prescription data only represent around half of total drug use in the elderly (patients aged 65 years and older).

Table 9.1. Drug Issuance Within Age Group

Issuance	Age Group (Percentage)					Total
	0–44	45–54	55–64	65–74	75+	
Prescription	62	61	59	53	47	58
Hospital order	11	19	24	32	41	20
Administered	11	9	7	6	4	9
Sample	5	4	4	4	3	4
Recommended	5	2	2	2	2	4
Stock dispensed	4	3	3	3	2	3
Sample and Rx	1	1	1	1	1	1
Total	100	100	100	100	100	100

Source: *National Disease and Therapeutic Index*, IMS America, Ltd, 1982.

NDTI data were used to generate a list of the 15 drug categories (as defined by the Uniform System of Classification, or USC) that were most frequently prescribed for patients aged 45 years and older to identify the ranks of these drug categories within each age group and to estimate the percentage of total prescriptions and prescriptions for each category that were written for patients in each age group.

To estimate overall outpatient drug exposure for an age group, the percentage of NDTI prescriptions accounted for by that age group was multiplied by the total number of prescriptions reported in the NPA and the result was adjusted for population size. Similar calculations were performed for the individual drug categories. For example, the NDTI indicated that 15.96% of beta-blocker prescriptions were written for people under 45 years of age, and the NPA reported that 52,265,000 beta-blocker prescriptions were dispensed from retail pharmacies in 1982. Multiplying these two figures resulted in an estimate of 8,341,000 beta-blocker prescriptions for people under 45 years of age and dividing this by the U.S. Census Bureau's population estimate for the group resulted in an average of 0.0526 prescriptions per person, or about 53 prescriptions/1,000 population/year.

The estimates of population exposure should be interpreted with caution because they were derived from two divergent data bases, each with its own set of inherent limitations and standard errors. They only represent outpatient prescription drug use and do not include prescriptions dispensed from outlets other than retail pharmacies. The estimates are probably most useful for making comparisons between age groups and between drug categories.

RESULTS

Although the percentage of total drug use accounted for by prescription issuance decreases with increasing age, the mean *number* of prescriptions per person per year increases regularly with age. People under 45 years of age had an average of about 4.6 prescriptions filled at retail pharmacies in 1982. People from 45 to 54 years of age received an average of approximately 6.9 prescriptions per person, people aged 55 to 64 got about 9.3, people 65 to 74 received about 13.6, and people 75 and older averaged about 16.9 prescriptions per person per year.

Table 9.2 lists the USC drug categories most frequently prescribed for patients aged 45 years and older. Systemic antiarthritics are the most commonly used, followed by beta-blockers, thiazide and related diuretics, and so on. Not surprisingly, drugs used in cardiovascular therapy are used frequently in this age group and ranked as numbers 2 through 8.

Table 9.2. Rank Within Age Groups for Drug Categories
Used Most Often by People Aged 45 and Older

USC Category	Age Group				
	0–44	45–54	55–64	65–74	75+
Systemic antiarthritics	8	1	2	1	2
Beta-blockers	20	2	1	2	6
Thiazide and related diuretics	28	3	3	3	4
Digitalis preparations	99	34	9	4	1
Potassium-sparing diuretics	49	5	4	5	5
Other oral diuretics (eg, furosemide)	78	18	8	6	3
Other antihypertensives (eg, methyldopa)	73	8	5	8	8
Nitrite/nitrate coronary vasodilators	*	16	7	7	7
Benzodiazepine tranquilizers	14	4	6	10	12
Diabetes therapy, oral	100	17	11	9	9
Codeine and combinations, oral analgesics	10	6	9	15	16
Plain corticoids, oral	15	12	13	14	15
Xanthine bronchodilators	18	23	14	11	13
Diabetes therapy, insulin	56	19	12	12	21
Tricyclic and related antidepressants	17	7	15	20	27

Source: *National Disease and Therapeutic Index*, IMS America, Ltd, 1982.
*Not in top 100.

Table 9.2 also provides information on the rank of the drug categories within each age group. Most of the cardiovascular categories are not highly ranked among people under 45 years of age with only beta-blockers and thiazide diuretics appearing in the top 30 categories. Nitrite and nitrate coronary vasodilators and digitalis preparations show the greatest differences between age groups. Nitrites and nitrates do not rank in the top 100 in the youngest age group; they are 16th among patients aged 45 to 54, and are ranked 7th in all three age groups 55 and older. Digitalis preparations go from 99th to 1st.

Digitalis and "other oral diuretics" (mainly furosemide) are the only cardiovascular categories that show a consistent increase in rank with age. The rankings for thiazide diuretics, potassium-sparing diuretics, and "other antihypertensives" (mainly methyldopa) are remarkably similar across the four older age groups, and nitrites/nitrates have identical rankings for the three groups 55 and older. Beta-blockers drop in the rankings for the oldest group.

Use of the eight noncardiovascular categories that were ranked in the top 15 differs from the cardiovascular categories in that the former tend to be ranked highly in all age groups. Except for diabetes therapy — oral hypoglycemics and insulin — they all ranked in the top 20 for people under 45. They are widely used and are not what one would generally think of as "geriatric drugs" (with the possible exception of systemic antiarthritics, which still rank as number 8 in the youngest age group).

The rankings for oral hypoglycemics are very low in people under 45 and increase with increasing age, which is what one might expect. The pattern for CNS-active drugs is interesting, with ranks for benzodiazepine tranquilizers, codeine, and tricyclic antidepressants being highest in the 45 to 54 age group and falling with increasing age.

Rankings are useful for identifying the most frequently used drugs and assessing the use of one category relative to another, but they don't provide fully adequate information on age differences *within* a drug category. Table 9.3 shows the age distribution for each drug category (with figures percentaged on row totals). Combining the fourth and fifth columns of this table provides estimates of the percentage of each drug category used in the elderly (patients 65 and older). For example, 76% of all digitalis prescriptions were written for these patients, as were 64% of "other oral diuretics" and 59% of nitrite or nitrate coronary vasodilators. The elderly accounted for less than half of the prescriptions for the other cardiovascular drug categories, but not much less, with beta-blockers representing the minimum of 38% use by the elderly. The greatest change in the cardiovascular market comes between the 45 to 54 group and the 55 to 64 group, with all seven drug categories increasing by at least 10 percentage points. Only digitalis and "other oral diuretics" show comparable increases in the 65 to 74 group, and they are also the only cardiovascular drugs that do not show a decreased market share for patients 75 years and older.

The age distribution of use within the noncardiovascular drug categories indicates again that a substantial portion of use for most of these categories is in the younger age group. The elderly (patients 65 years and older) represent a majority of the market only in the case of oral diabetes therapy. They account for around 39% of insulin therapy and only about one-third of systemic antiarthritic prescriptions. Looking at only market share, it could be

Table 9.3. Age Distribution of Drug Mentions Within Drug Category

USC Category	Age Group (Percentage)					
	0–44	45–54	55–64	65–74	75 +	Total
Systemic antiarthritics	29	15	21	20	14	100
Beta-blockers	16	18	29	25	13	100
Thiazide and related diuretics	14	16	26	26	18	100
Digitalis preparations	4	5	16	32	44	100
Potassium-sparing diuretics	12	16	26	25	21	100
Other oral diuretics (eg, furosemide)	8	8	20	30	34	100
Other antihypertensives (eg, methyldopa)	10	15	29	28	19	100
Nitrite/nitrate coronary vasodilators	4	11	26	32	27	100
Benzodiazepine tranquilizers	40	19	19	14	8	100
Diabetes therapy, oral	6	13	27	33	21	100
Codeine and combinations, oral analgesics	53	14	15	11	7	100
Plain corticoids, oral	44	13	16	17	9	100
Xanthine bronchodilators	43	9	17	20	11	100
Diabetes therapy, insulin	22	14	25	27	12	100
Tricyclic and related antidepressants	46	19	17	12	6	100

Source: *National Disease and Therapeutic Index*, IMS America Ltd, 1982.

said that diabetes therapy is more "geriatric" than antiarthritics. For all of these categories, as with most of the cardiovascular drugs, people 75 and over account for a lower percentage of drug use than do people from 65 to 74 years old. One obvious explanation for the lower market shares in the oldest group is simply that there are fewer people in this age group and these data do not take population size into account. They also provide no information on the actual quantity of the drug being used.

From a public health perspective we are most interested in population exposure: how many people are taking how much of a given type of drug. Unfortunately, we don't have a population-based survey that is done yearly, that covers all drugs, and that is done on a national level. We do have ongoing comprehensive data from the NPA that provide us with national estimates of the number of prescriptions dispensed from retail pharmacies. In the absence of data on "number of people," we generally use "number of prescriptions" as an indicator of population exposure. Estimates of outpatient population exposure derived from NPA, NDTI, and U.S. Bureau of the Census figures are presented in Table 9.4. As discussed in the Methods section, these are not hard and fast numbers, but represent our best estimates of age differences in drug exposure. Data are limited to prescriptions only, and the percent of total drug use accounted for by prescriptions decreases with increasing age.

Looking first at the cardiovascular drug categories, these data indicate that beta-blocker use does decrease in the 75 years and over group, but they do not show the decreasing use for thiazide and potassium-sparing diuretics,

Table 9.4. Prescriptions*/1,000 Population/Year

USC Category	Age Group				
	0–44	45–54	55–64	65–74	75+
Systemic antiarthritics	113	419	590	747	785
Beta-blockers	53	415	676	800	638
Thiazide and related diuretics	36	295	496	679	693
Digitalis preparations	6	56	191	521	1071
Potassium-sparing diuretics	31	281	460	628	774
Other oral diuretics (eg, furosemide)	15	106	249	521	880
Other antihypertensives (eg, methyldopa)	18	194	371	495	501
Nitrite/nitrate coronary vasodilators	7	140	348	589	739
Benzodiazepine tranquilizers	144	491	488	494	420
Diabetes therapy, oral	7	98	201	340	327
Codeine and combinations, oral analgesics	199	371	411	407	368
Plain corticoids, oral	42	86	111	156	132
Xanthine bronchodilators	60	87	170	276	231
Diabetes therapy, insulin	14	63	112	164	113
Tricyclic and related antidepressants	54	160	145	136	114

Based on data from the *National Disease and Therapeutic Index* and the *National Prescription Audit*, IMS America, Ltd, 1982.

*Only prescriptions dispensed from retail pharmacies.

"other antihypertensives," and nitrite and nitrate coronary vasodilators that was indicated by the market-share data in Table 9.3. The two drug categories that did show an increased percentage of use in the oldest group showed an enormous increase in exposure. People aged 75 years and older use over twice as much digitalis as people between 65 and 74 years old and about 19 times as much as people aged 45 to 54. They receive about 69% more prescriptions in the "other oral diuretic" category than the 65 to 74 age group, and about eight times as many as the 45 to 54 group.

The greatest relative increase in the utilization of beta-blockers, thiazide and related diuretics, potassium-sparing diuretics, and "other antihypertensives" occurs before the age of 65. Leaving aside the 0 to 44 age group, which is not really a fair comparison because it is so broad, the greatest increase in the use of these four drug categories is in the 55 to 64 group.

Among the noncardiovascular drug categories listed in Table 9.4, systemic antiarthritics are the only drugs for which exposure increases for each successive age group, including the 75 and older group. The elderly account for only one-third of all systemic antiarthritic prescriptions, but their exposure to this drug class is extensive due to the large number of prescriptions dispensed for such products (a total of over 60 million in 1982, or 4% of all prescriptions).

Exposure to the other noncardiovascular categories decreases in people 75 and over. Use of oral corticoids, xanthine bronchodilators, and diabetes therapy (both oral hypoglycemics and insulin) increases with age up through the 65 to 74 group then decreases in the oldest group. Use of benzodiazepine tranquilizers is fairly comparable in the three groups between 45 to 74, whereas tricyclic exposure peaks in patients aged 45 to 54 and decreases in each successive age group. Analgesic codeine use is highest in the 55 to 64 group but is very similar to use by people 65 to 74 years old.

It should be noted at this point that ranking drug categories by prescriptions per 1,000 people will give results that are very similar but not identical to previous rankings based solely on NDTI prescriptions (eg, systemic antiarthritics were ranked as number 2 in the 75 and older group based on NDTI alone, but these patients receive more prescriptions for both digitalis preparations and "other oral diuretics" than for systemic antiarthritics). These minor discrepancies probably relate to the fact that NDTI data come from a physician panel, where a prescription with three refills would be counted as one drug report, whereas NPA pharmacy data would indicate four prescriptions.

In summary, the drugs most frequently prescribed to people aged 45 years and older fall into three basic groups: cardiovascular drugs, diabetes therapy, and drugs that are in wide general use (that is, used relatively frequently by the younger population as well).

DISCUSSION

The use of 15 different drug categories was reviewed from three different perspectives. First, the categories were ranked within each age group, which identified the most frequently used drugs and provided some idea of their use relative to one another. The second framework considered the age distributions within each drug category to characterize the population currently getting the drugs that are on the market now. The third type of data — prescriptions/1,000 population/year — is the most useful for estimating population drug exposure because it takes population size and prescription volume into account. Unfortunately, it is also the "fuzziest" and the most time consuming to calculate.

Data generally indicated that use of systemic antiarthritics and all cardiovascular categories except beta-blockers increases regularly with age but that the greatest increase in use of these drugs often comes before the age of 65. In fact, nitrites/nitrates were the only cardiovascular drugs whose greatest increase occurred in the 65 to 74 group. Two categories, digitalis preparations and "other oral diuretics," increased the most in patients aged 75 and older, and use of systemic antiarthritics and the remaining four cardiovascular categories increased the most in patients aged 55 to 64. Patterns were more variable for the other drug categories. Exposure to antidiabetic drugs and five noncardiovascular drug categories decreased in the older group (people aged 75 and older). These drugs were more likely than cardiovascular drugs to have their greatest increase in exposure in the 65 to 74 group.

Chapter 10

ADVERSE DRUG REACTION SURVEILLANCE IN THE GERIATRIC POPULATION: A PRELIMINARY VIEW

Steven R. Moore, RPH, MPH

Judith K. Jones, MD, PhD

The untoward effects of prescription drugs remain a major concern among elderly patients. In addition to such effects as the lack of efficacy and potentiation of other drug effects, the occurrence of adverse drug reactions (ADRs) is of major consequence to the elderly. Not only can adverse drug reactions prevent a cure or amelioration of an existing physical condition, but ADRs can also create new iatrogenic conditions and affect mobility and lifestyle in addition to being the causative factor in accidents or mental confusion. Besides the obvious harmful effect to the individual, society shares the detrimental effect in the cost of medical and domiciliary care to affected elderly individuals. Indirectly, lost productivity of impaired elderly individuals creates further societal costs.

With an increasingly older population, the absolute number of ADR incidents is likely to increase. Additionally, multiple drug use by the older consumer creates a situation where more ADRs can be expected, compounding the problem. Thus, the nature and the effect of ADRs in the elderly population can have a much greater impact than comparable ADRs in the general or younger population.

The knowledge of ADRs in this country is an integral component to the ongoing regulation of the safety and efficacy of drugs by the Food and Drug

The opinions expressed in this paper are solely those of the authors. Special thanks for aid in the management of the data for this paper is extended to Fred Wegner and Judy Brown of the American Association of Retired Persons and pharmacists Peter Garofalo, Henry Peters, Paul Reznek, Lou Rubenstein, and Paul Woods.

Administration (FDA). Since the early 1960s, the FDA has collected spontaneous reports of suspected ADRs. Since 1969, the FDA has computerized these reports and maintains probably the largest data base on ADRs in the world. The FDA is mandated by regulation (21 CFR 310, 301) to require the pharmaceutical industry to submit reports of suspected or known ADRs for their marketed drugs. These submissions account for about 80% of all reports received by the FDA. Purely spontaneous reports from the medical and health professions and consumers account for the other 20% of the reports in this data base. The cumulative data file has almost 200,000 ADR reports. In addition to submitted data, literature and adverse drug reaction registries (hepatic, ophthalmic, and dermatologic) provide additional ADRs. Besides internal use for analysis of changes in labeling and the preparation of various scientific and medical publications, the data base is used extensively by private sector entities through the Freedom of Information Act. A number of previous reports provide detailed descriptions of the system.[1-4].

The formal mechanism for reporting suspected and known ADRs is FDA Form 1639, (Figure 10.1) titled Drug Experience Report. Besides the characteristics of the patient, the reaction (ie, experience), suspected drug, other drugs used concommitantly, and any pertinent medical or physical facts are also included in the report. Upon receipt by the FDA, reports are evaluated, sorted, and categorized by drug type, seriousness, and presence or absence of a similar reaction in the current drug labeling. For administrative clarity, reports are classified as to causality using an established causality algorithm. Reports that are serious, new, or highly associated with the drug (according to the algorithm) are given higher priority for analysis. All reports are entered into the computerized data base after undergoing the above analysis. As demonstrated by Form 1639, the causality algorithm, and the medical evaluation, all drugs with even a temporal association with the reported ADR will enter the system and be recorded for the respective drug and the respective reaction. Thus, drugs that may have very little probability of actually precipitating a reaction may be linked to the reaction due to their temporal association with a causative drug. Similarly, a drug that does not appear on first viewing to have a relationship to a particular reaction may actually have a relationship upon retrospective analysis with a large enough sampling of similar reactions.

With such a data base, both positive and negative factors related to its effectiveness must be considered. On the positive side, the mere size of the data base and the number of reported reactions suggest its potential to sample the actual experience with adverse drug reactions over time. Additionally, the ability to characterize the reports by age and sex, and sometimes other characteristics, allows use of this data for better understanding of the qualitative nature of drug toxicity.

There are also certain limitations to the data base. Foremost, the system is a spontaneous system and the rigor of a controlled study is simply not

DEPARTMENT OF HEALTH AND HUMAN SERVICES PUBLIC HEALTH SERVICE FOOD AND DRUG ADMINISTRATION ROCKVILLE˙ MD 20857	*FORM APPROVED: OMB NO. 0910-0002* *Use of this form is prohibited after 12/31/84.*

DRUG EXPERIENCE REPORT   FDA CONTROL NO.   ACCESSION NO. ☐☐☐☐☐☐☐☐☐☐☐☐

I.   REACTION INFORMATION

1. PATIENT ID/INITIALS (In Confidence)	2. AGE	3. SEX	4. WGT.	5. HT.	6. REPORTING DATE			7. REACTION ONSET DATE		
					MO	DA	YR	MO	DA	YR

8. DESCRIBE SUSPECTED REACTION(S)

9. OUTCOME OF REACTION TO DATE
☐ Alive with sequelae
☐ Recovered
☐ Still under treatment for reaction
☐ Died (Give cause/date)

10. TESTS/LABORATORY DATA CONFIRMING REACTION (Include biopsy and/or autopsy results)

11. WAS OUTPATIENT TREATMENT FOR REACTION REQUIRED? ☐ Yes ☐ No

12. WAS HOSPITAL TREATMENT FOR REACTION REQUIRED? ☐ Yes ☐ No

II.   SUSPECT DRUG(S) INFORMATION

13. SUSPECT DRUG(S) - TRADE/GENERIC NAME(S), MANUFACTURER, IND/NDA NO.

14. TOTAL DAILY DOSE

15. ROUTE OF ADMINISTRATION

16. INDICATION(S) FOR USE	17. THERAPY DATES *(From/To)*	18. THERAPY DURATION

19a. WAS TREATMENT WITH SUSPECTED DRUG REDUCED IN DOSAGE? ☐ Yes ☐ No OR: ☐ Discontinued	19b. DID REACTION ABATE? ☐ Yes ☐ No	20a. WAS DRUG REINTRODUCED OR DOSE INCREASED? ☐ Yes ☐ No	20b. DID REACTION REAPPEAR? ☐ Yes ☐ No

III.   RECENT/CONCOMITANT DRUGS AND MEDICAL PROBLEMS

21. OTHER DRUGS	TOTAL DAILY DOSE	ROUTE	DATES/DURATION OF ADMINISTRATION	INDICATIONS

22. DESCRIBE OTHER RELEVANT MEDICAL HISTORY (i.e., allergies, environmental or occupational exposure, previous drug reactions, pregnancy with gravidity/parity, ethnic origin.)

Your cooperation is needed to insure comprehensive, accurate, and timely use and interpretation of these data.

23. MFR NAME/ADDRESS	24. Check one ☐ Initial Report ☐ Follow-up Report	25. REPORTER'S NAME AND ADDRESS (In confidence)
MFR CONTROL NO. DATE SENT TO FDA		

NOTE: *Required of manufacturers by 21 CFR 310.300, 310.301 and 431.60. Manufacturers may attach additional clinical material and product analyses at their discretion.*

26. MAY THE SOURCE OF THIS REPORT BE RELEASED TO THE ARMED FORCES INSTITUTE OF PATHOLOGY? ☐ Yes ☐ No

FORM FDA 1639 (1/82) PREVIOUS EDITIONS ARE OBSOLETE.

Figure 10.1.

present. Next, the system is the result of some 15 years of reports for drugs whose clinical and demographic use may vary over time, and the reports can reflect this. Third, given that the reports are spontaneous, public awareness (ie, via the press) may create periodic "bandwagon" effects in reporting. Fourth, over-the-counter drugs have limited representation in the system and often are in the system due to concurrent use with prescription drugs. Fifth, the nature of the reporting form creates certain data that are put into the system, but this may or may not be meaningful for certain questions. Sixth, the reports of adverse effects often decrease after labeling reflects expected reactions, even if the same adverse reactions continue to occur. Finally, multiple other factors such as the lack of completeness of the reports, the lack of ability to get further information on a number of reports, and multiple source reporting of adverse effects require that use of the system's data take these limitations into account. It is for this reason that the major use of the system is to "signal" certain problems and suggest trends that might be verified in more controlled data resources.

Given the existence of the ADR data base and the concern that special population groups (in this case the elderly) may need special study, the opportunity to study ADRs in geriatrics was present. The American Association of Retired Persons kindly provides technical assistance, including the services of five retired pharmacists to undertake this activity.

Initially a printout for the entire data base (1968 to 1982), with all reported adverse drug reactions grouped by pharmacologic class (Table 10.1), was obtained. The initial tally provided the ranking of the classes with the highest number of reported ADR terms reported for the entire population over 13 years (1968 to 1982). A subsequent tally provided a similar ranking for the pharmacologic classes with the highest reported number of ADR terms for the elderly population (set arbitrarily at 65 years of age and over) (Table 10.2). For the top 13 pharmacologic classes with the highest number of reports of geriatric ADRs, the top five generic drugs for each class were determined and characterized by the number of ADR terms, number of terms by body system, age grouping of the patients, and finally the sex of the patient (Table 10.3). This analysis excluded any ADRs with unknown age values, and only ADRs occurring in the geriatric age groups were thus tabulated.

Table 10.1. Total Adverse Drug Reaction Occurrence (through FY 1983)

Rank	Pharmacologic Class	ADR Occurrence
1	Antibiotics	33,959
2	Tranquilizers	33,720
3	Antiparkinsonian	17,587
4	Narcotic/analgesic	15,471
5	Anticonvulsants	12,721
6	Antiarthritics	11,940
7	Antineoplastic	11,881
8	Diuretics	11,658
9	Analgesics/antipyretics	11,065
10	Radiographic	10,772
11	Antidepressants	10,428
12	Antihypertensives	9,997
13	Antiarrhythmics	9,086
14	Sedatives/hypnotics	7,105

Table 10.2. Most Frequently Occurring ADRs in Geriatric Age Group (through FY 1983)

Rank	Pharmacologic Class	ADR Terms	% Over 65 of Total ADR in Class	Rank of Total ADR in Class
1	Antiparkinsonian	8986	53.4	1
2	Antibiotics	5709	22	8
3	Antiarthritics	3169	27	7
4	Antiarrhythmics	3118	34	5
5	Diuretics	3019	35	4
6	Tranquilizers	2369	7	12
7	Antihypertensives	2200	31	6
8	Analgesics/antipyretics	1346	15.5	10
9	Antidepressants	1234	12	11
10	Radiographic	1105	21	9
11	Adrenergic blocking agents	945	43.6	3
12	Anticonvulsants	843	6.9	13
13	Vasodilators	811	49	2

The resulting data present a variety of potential areas for further investigation. Of primary concern is the occurrence of a large quantity of ADR reports where the use of the drug is relatively low. Drugs that particularly affect one sex or one age group are also of concern and such findings may support unique populations at high risk. Drugs that affect body systems in the elderly differently than in the general population also present territory for further investigation. See Table 10.4 for a list of body system classifications. At the present time, only the preliminary tabulation of ADR terms within the various generic entities, pharmacologic classes, and demographic boundaries has been completed.

Future areas for emphasis may well result in descriptions of some certain possible risk factors for elderly populations. It would be best if ADRs can be compared with population exposure. Unfortunately, a satisfactory estimate for 13 cumulative years is not available. However, as a crude surrogate, we examined one approach. The numerator for the ADR exposure is the total number of ADR terms in the system for the generic drug entity. The denominator, admittedly skewed to newer drugs, is the number of drug mentions in the National Disease and Therapeutic Index survey for fiscal year 1983. The higher the ratio, theoretically the greater the risk of an ADR occurring (Table 10.5).

With the aging of our population, the increased use of newer and more potent drugs within the elderly population, and the increasing sophistication of postmarketing surveillance tools, the ability to know and hopefully reduce both the occurrence and severity of adverse drug reactions in the elderly population is a challenge that has drawn increasing attention.

Table 10.3. Most Frequently Reported Generic Drugs Within Each Class

Drug Class: Antiparkinsonian			Drug Class: Antibiotics		
Drug	Total ADR Terms	Rank	Drug	Total ADR Terms	Rank
Levodopa	6949	1	Ampicillin	726	1
Trihexyphenidyl	511	2	Tobramycin	580	2
Carbidopa-levidopa			Cephalothin	487	3
(Sinemet)	261	3	Clindamycin	474	4
Benztropine mesylate	209	4	Gentamycin	369	5
Amantadine	191	5			
Predominate body systems:	Metabolic and nutritional (28%) Hemic and lymphatic (26%) Nervous (17%)		Predominate body systems:	Metabolic and nutritional (22.8%) Skin and appendages (22.5%) Digestive (19.8%)	
Predominate age group:	65–74 (65%)		Predominate age group:	65–74 (53.6%)	
Predominate sex:	Male (78%)		Predominate sex:	Male (54%)	

• •

Drug Class: Antiarthritics			Drug Class: Antiarrhythmics		
Drug	Total ADR Terms	Rank	Drug	Total ADR Terms	Rank
Sulindac	1073	1	Digoxin	1552	1
Benoxaprofen	757	2	Propranolol	765	2
Ibuprofen	667	3	Procainamide	467	3
Piroxicam	539	4	Disopyramide	292	4
Indomethacin	537	5	Verapamil	238	5
Predominate body systems:	Digestive (27.3%) Hemic and lymphatic (12.1%) Skin and appendages (11.0%)		Predominate body systems:	Cardiovascular (21%) Nervous (14%) Body as a whole (13.5%) Digestive (13.2%)	
Predominate age group:	65–74 (56.3%)		Predominate age group:	65–74 (57.7%)	
Predominate sex:	Female (69.6%)		Predominate sex:	Neither	

• •

Drug Class: Diuretics			Drug Class: Tranquilizers		
Drug	Total ADR Terms	Rank	Drug	Total ADR Terms	Rank
Hydrochlorothiazide	1702	1	Diazepam	627	1
Furosemide	1112	2	Chlorpromazine	234	2
Triamterene	704	3	Haloperidol	216	3
Selacryn	355	4	Hydroxyzine	90	4
Spironolactone	340	5	Doxepin	46	5
Predominate body systems:	Digestive (16.5%) Metabolic and nutritional (14%) Hemic and lymphatic (12.3%)		Predominate body systems:	Nervous (30%) Digestive (12.6%) Hemic and lymphatic (11%)	
Predominate age group:	65–74 (59.6%)		Predominate age group:	65–74 (56%)	
Predominate sex:	Female (52.8%)		Predominate sex:	Female (56%)	

• •

Table 10.3 continued

Drug Class: Antihypertensives		
Drug	Total ADR Terms	Rank
Methyldopa	1078	1
Hydrochlorothiazide	371	2
Reserpine	322	3
Hydralazine	316	4
Prazosin	240	5
Predominate body systems:	Hemic and lymphatic (18.1%) Digestive (15%) Nervous (14.2%)	
Predominate age group:	65–74 (65.4%)	
Predominate sex:	Female (63.8%)	

Drug Class: Analgesics/Antipyretics		
Drug	Total ADR Terms	Rank
Aspirin	530	1
Zomepirac	507	2
Acetaminophen	355	3
Propoxyphene	265	4
Pentazocine	250	5
Predominate body systems:	Digestive (19.5%) Nervous (16%)	
Predominate age group:	65–74 (61.8%)	
Predominate sex:	Female (64.4%)	

• •

Drug Class: Antidepressants		
Drug	Total ADR Terms	Rank
Imipramine	395	1
Amitriptyline	307	2
Trazodone	213	3
Doxepin	62	4
Nortriptyline	26	5
Predominate body systems:	Nervous (38%)	
Predominate age group:	65–74 (68%)	
Predominate sex:	Female (59%)	

Drug Class: Radiographic		
Drug	Total ADR Terms	Rank
Diatrizoate meglumine	638	1
Diatrizoate sodium	592	2
Iothalamate meglumine	212	3
Iothalamate sodium	146	4
Iodipamide methyl glucamide	53	5
Predominate body systems:	Cardiovascular (30%) Body as a whole (19.7%) Respiratory (14.9%)	
Predominate age group:	65–74 (63%)	
Predominate sex:	Male (59%)	

• •

Drug Class: Adrenergic Blocking Agents		
Drug	Total ADR Terms	Rank
Timolol	543	1
Atenolol	293	2
Metaprolol	242	3
Ergoloid mesylates (Hydergine)	192	4
Nadalol	91	5
Predominate body systems:	Cardiovascular (20%) Nervous (19.2%) Special senses (12.3%)	
Predominate age group:	65–74 (61.4%)	
Predominate sex:	Female (59%)	

Drug Class: Anticonvulsants		
Drug	Total ADR Terms	Rank
Phenytoin	249	1
Carbamazepine	160	2
Valproic acid	26	3
Primidone	12	4
Mephenytoin	4	5
Predominate body systems:	Nervous (20.6%) Skin and appendages (14.9%) Hemic and lymphatic (13.3%) Body as a whole (12.4%)	
Predominate age group:	65–74 (59.6%)	
Predominate sex:	Female (57.2%)	

Drug Class: Vasodilators		
Drug	Total ADR Terms	Rank
Isosorbide dinitrate	312	1
Nitroglycerin	267	2
Verapamil	154	3
Dipyridamole	146	4
Papaverine	70	5
Predominate body systems:	Cardiovascular (16.3%) Body as a whole (15.3%) Digestive (14.5%) Nervous (13.8%)	
Predominate age group:	65–74 (56.7%)	
Predominate sex:	None	

Table 10.4. Body System Classifications for ADRs

Body as a Whole
Cardiovascular
Digestive
Endocrine
Hemic and Lymphatic
Metabolic and Nutritional
Musculoskeletal
Nervous
Respiratory
Skin and Appendages
Special Senses
Urogenital

Table 10.5. Ratio of ADR Terms to Drug Mentions For Selected Drugs

Drug	Ratio ($\times 10^5$)	Rank
Dipyridamole	4	1
Atenolol	18	2
Timolol	18	2
Ibuprofen	25	3
Piroxicam	26	4
Diazepam	29	5
Indomethacin	30	6
Amantadine	59	7
Carbamazepine	64	8
Sulindac	76	9
Benztropine	106	10
Cephalothin	107	11
Trihexyphenidyl	207	12
Tobramycin	282	13

REFERENCES

1. Jones JK: Suspected drug induced hepatic reactions reported to the FDA adverse reaction system: An overview. *Semin Liver Dis* 1982; 1(2):157–167.

2. Jones JK: Adverse drug reactions in the community health setting: Approaches to recognizing, counseling, and reporting. *Family Community Health* 1982; 8:58–67.

3. Lee B, Turner W: Food and drug administration's adverse drug reaction monitoring program. *Am J Hosp Pharm* 1978; 25:929,932.

4. Pearson K: The pharmacist and adverse reaction reporting. *Hosp Pharm* 1982; 17:421–430.

Chapter 11

DRUG UTILIZATION IN THE RURAL ELDERLY: PERSPECTIVES FROM A POPULATION STUDY

Robert B. Wallace, MD

This paper presents preliminary results of the kinds of information concerning drug utilization in the elderly that might be obtained from community-based population surveys. There are several reasons why this is an important perspective. It is the most direct method of measuring drug utilization behavior; it allows the study of over-the-counter as well as prescribed medications; it allows the correlation of drug behavior with other health characteristics and habits; and finally, it defines the population impact of drug utilization problems and allows generation of hypotheses for predicting who will have these problems and how to prevent them.

Our study is one of three, along with similar investigations at Harvard and Yale Universities, that is sponsored by the National Institute on Aging, collectively forming the "Established Populations for Epidemiologic Study of the Elderly." Our own study was specifically designed to explore a broad range of physical, mental, and social characteristics of the rural elderly. The target population was persons 65 years and older living in two rural counties adjacent to the county in which the University of Iowa is located. Of the target population 3,673, or 80%, were interviewed. Fifteen percent of these subjects had abbreviated, telephone, or surrogate interviews, either because of refusal for the full interview or intercurrent illness. Thus, the data are from the 3,096 persons who were interviewed in the home, two-thirds of whom were women.

The initial baseline survey took place between December 1981, and July 1982. Along with other information, we took a detailed drug utilization history with the interviewers asking to see all medication containers for both legend and over-the-counter drugs. In cases where prescribing information or drug identity could not be obtained, calls were made to pharmacies and physician offices. Entries for legend drugs were coded by the Drug Product Information coding system. We established our own coding system for over-the-counter drugs, in an analogous format. After the initial interview, we have been doing annual follow-up interviews by telephone. The second annual follow-up is currently underway. It must be emphasized again that the data are preliminary and presented only to explore the kinds of information available.

The first set of tables deals with the general utilization of drugs in our entire elderly population, based on the initial survey. Table 11.1 shows the general therapeutic categories for legend drugs used. They are dominated first by cardiovascular and second by central nervous system agents. Table 11.2 shows the distribution of doses for those medications prescribed on a daily basis. Nearly 40% of the drugs were to be taken only once per day. Nearly 20% of the drugs were prescribed to be taken four or more times per day. Table 11.3 shows the distribution of dosage forms. This was overwhelmingly dominated by tablets and capsules. Table 11.4 shows where the prescriptions were dispensed. I was somewhat surprised that 9% of the prescriptions were being dispensed by physicians. I don't know whether this is peculiar to our own rural areas or a more general phenomenon. Please also note that nearly 14% of the subjects had drugs from multiple pharmacies. This obviously adds to the problem of monitoring drug interactions.

Table 11.1. Distribution of Legend Drug Categories

Category	Percentage
Antiinfectives	3.2
CNS agents	21.2
Cardiovascular	50.8
Hormones	6.5
Blood formation	2.0
GI agents	4.7
Miscellaneous	11.6

Table 11.2. Number of Daily Doses

Daily Doses	Percentage
As directed	8.7
½ dose	2.1
1	38.2
1½	0.5
2	21.2
3	11.4
4	11.6
5+	6.3

Table 11.3. Dosage Forms

Dosage Form	Percentage
Oral tablets	77.6
Oral capsules	14.4
Oral liquid	0.8
Topical cream	0.6
Nonophthal. liquid	0.6
Ophthal. liquid	1.1
Vaginal suppository	0.1
Inhalents	0.4
Rectal suppository/misc.	4.4

Table 11.4. Dispenser of Prescription

Dispenser	Percentage
Physician	9.2
Single source pharmacy	68.8
Multiple source pharmacy	13.7
Not specified	8.3

Table 11.5 shows that a wide variety of dosing schedules were prescribed. It is of interest that over half of the drugs were prescribed on a more complicated schedule than a daily basis, either requiring PRN use, tablet-splitting, alternate day and holiday use, or combinations of these schedules. These more complicated dosage schedules require a certain amount of manual dexterity and mental function. This could serve as a sign of potential problems in drug use that may arise in this elderly population.

Table 11.5. Dosing Schedule

Dosing Schedule	Percentage
PRN	15.1
Scheduled daily	41.3
Tablet splitting	25.4
Alternate day	22.1
Tablet splitting + alternate day/holiday dosing	7.3
Tablet splitting + PRN	0.2

Table 11.6 shows the distribution of the number of drugs used per person among those reporting any drug use. Forty percent of this population reported the use of three or more drugs, and 10% the use of five or more drugs. Table 11.7 shows the distribution of the categories of over-the-counter drugs. This is dominated by analgesics and antipyretics, multivitamins, and laxatives, in that order. Table 11.8 looks at the top 10 mentions of over-the-counter drugs. This again is dominated by aspirin-containing drugs and by nutritional supplements. Parenthetically, enough of the population are using specific supplements such as vitamin C and vitamin E to the point where one can actually do prospective epidemiologic studies of their impact on the more common incident diseases. Table 11.9 shows the mean number of drugs reportedly used in a one-day period. One can see that the mean was slightly higher for over-the-counter than for legend drugs. This suggests that in considering drug interactions, complications, or costs, there must be close consideration of over-the-counter products. Table 11.10 shows the percentage reportedly consuming any psychoactive drug over the 2 weeks prior to interview. For both men and women this was nearly 10% of the population.

Table 11.6. Distribution of Number of Drugs per Respondent Among Those Reporting Any Drug Use (Legend and OTC)

No. of Drugs	Percentage of Persons
1	37.3
2	22.8
3	14.5
4	11.4
5	6.0
6	4.2
7	2.1
8	1.7

Table 11.7. Ranking of Over-the-Counter Drugs by Therapeutic Category

Therapeutic Category	Percentage
Analgesics and antipyretics	40.3
Multivitamins	28.7
Laxatives	12.9
Antacids	6.5
Diet supplements	3.2
Topical decongestants and cold products	2.2
Antitussives	0.9
Dermatologicals	0.6
Miscellaneous	4.7

Table 11.8. Top Ten Over-The-Counter Drugs (Mentions)

Drug	Percentage of all OTCs
Aspirin (unspecified)	12.9
Bufferin	7.8
Tylenol	6.8
Anacin	5.6
Vitamin C	5.3
Metamucil	4.2
Vitamin E	3.2
Multivitamin (unspecified)	3.1
Vitamin (unspecified)	2.2
Milk of Magnesia	2.1

Table 11.9. Mean Number of Drugs Reported Consumed in a One-Day Period per Respondent

Drug Category	Mean
Legend	1.21
Over-the-counter	1.35
Unknown (2.9%)	0.08
Total	2.64

Table 11.10. Percentage Reporting Psychoactive Drug Consumption — Two-Week Prevalence

Drug Category	Percentage	
	Male	Female
Antidepressant	2.3	2.6
Tranquilizer/sedative/hypnotic	7.0	7.1

The next few tables show the relationship between drug use and other health characteristics in our population. Table 11.11 shows the mean number of drugs according to self-perceived health status. As one can see, the worse the health status, the more drugs are used. This in itself is not surprising, but suggests that drug use can be used as a surrogate for health status in certain analytic activities. When self-perceived health status is compared to the use of over-the-counter drugs, as shown in Table 11.12, the gradient is by no means as strong in men and is actually not present in women. This opens up several avenues of research on the differences in the predictors of use of prescription versus over-the-counter drugs. Table 11.13 shows the use of legend drugs in men according to the presence of symptoms of depression. In this particular setting, there was essentially no excess use of drugs among those with depressive symptoms. Since there is always an added

Table 11.11. Mean Number of Legend Drugs Reportedly Consumed in a Two-Week Period According to Self-Perceived Health Status

	Mean Number Drugs	
Health Status	Males	Females
Excellent	1.8	1.9
Good	2.3	2.3
Fair	2.8	3.0
Poor	4.2	3.4

Table 11.12. Mean Number of OTC Drugs Reportedly Consumed in a Two-Week Period According to Self-Perceived Health Status

	Mean Number Drugs	
Health Status	Males	Females
Excellent	1.2	1.3
Good	1.3	1.3
Fair	1.4	1.4
Poor	1.8	1.4

Table 11.13. Mean Number of Legend Drugs
Reportedly Consumed in a Two-Week Period
According to the Presence of
Depressive Symptoms—Males

Age Group (years)	Mean Number Drugs	
	Depressive sx(+)	Depressive sx(−)
65–69	2.2	2.6
70–74	2.5	3.0
75–79	2.2	2.9
80 +	2.5	2.7

potential problem in cross-sectional data of discerning cause and effect, it would be hard to judge any drug use/depression relationship that emerges. Because there is sometimes a potential interaction in the metabolism of drugs and alcohol, we look at the mean number of drugs according to the use or nonuse of liquor at least once a week, shown in Table 11.14. As one can see, there were no great differences in either sex for mean drug use according to whether or not liquor was also consumed, and in some of the female age categories there was actually greater mean drug use among those reporting liquor consumption.

The final few tables show preliminary results from a pilot effort at detecting adverse drug reactions in the second annual telephone follow-up of our population, which is now in progress. Table 11.15 shows that over 10% of the entire population in the pilot survey reported an adverse drug reaction in the year prior to the survey. In these 50 reactions, of which 49 were attributed to legend drugs, the most frequent category was related to gastrointestinal upset, followed by perceived personality change and syncope. Table 11.16 shows the therapeutic categories to which each adverse drug reaction was attributed. This list was dominated by hypotensive and diuretic drugs fol-

Table 11.14. Mean Number of Legend Drugs Reportedly Taken
According to Use of Liquor (at least once per week)

Age Group (years)	Mean Number Drugs			
	Males		Females	
	Liq (−)	Liq (+)	Liq (−)	Liq (+)
65–69	2.4	2.0	2.2	2.6
70–74	2.5	1.9	2.5	2.4
75–79	2.6	1.8	2.4	3.0

lowed by perceived personality change and syncope. Table 11.16 shows the therapeutic categories to which each adverse drug reaction was attributed. This list was dominated by hypotensive and diuretic drugs followed by the analgesics and antipyretics. This generally mirrors the prevalence of use of these agents in the population. Finally, we looked at some of the medical system utilization responses to these reported adverse reactions, as shown in Table 11.17. Of the 50 subjects reporting reactions, 92% consulted their physician. In 42% of the instances, this led to the ordering of one or more laboratory tests, and in 62% of the times the drug indicated was stopped. Thus it appears that these reactions could potentially lead to considerable use of medical resources. We are currently exploring the possibility of characterizing the risk profiles of those subjects more likely to report an adverse drug reaction.

Table 11.15. Community Survey* of Noninstitutional Adverse Drug Reactions

Adverse Drug Reaction	Percentage
Nausea, vomiting, epigastric pain	13
Personality change	6
Syncope	6
Weakness, malaise, somnolence	5
Dry mouth	5
Tremor	4
Rash	4
Urinary retention	2
Diarrhea	2
Numb extremities	2

*50/482 subjects = 10.4%.

Table 11.16. Therapeutic Category of Drugs with Attributed Adverse Reactions

Therapeutic Category	No. Adverse Reactions
Hypotensive/diuretic	14
Analgesic/antipyretic	7
Cardiac	5
Autonomic	5
Antiinfective	4
Psychotherapeutic	3
Hormones	3
Unknown	3

Table 11.17. Responses to Drug Reaction

Response	Percentage
Patient consulted physician	92
Laboratory test(s) ordered	42
Drug consumption stopped	62

In summary, we feel that population surveys offer information that is complementary to that obtained by the other means, and in some instances offer information garnered by no other means. Some of these areas are only now being explored, and there is much work yet to do in determining the reliability and validity of the data being collected. However, there is considerable promise in the population approach to drug use in the elderly.

Chapter 12

GERIATRIC DRUG EPIDEMIOLOGY AND HEALTH SERVICES RESEARCH BASED ON LARGE-SCALE COMPUTERIZED DATA SETS

Jerry Avorn, MD

It is well known that the elderly are at increased risk of adverse drug reactions for a wide number of reasons. These include diminished hepatic metabolism and renal excretion of ingested drugs, changes in receptor sensitivity for many commonly used drug categories, changes in body composition affecting the volume of distribution of drugs, and several other changes that are known to occur as part of the aging process itself.[1,2] In addition, because of the increased number of coexisting illnesses and therapies in many elderly patients, risks from drug-disease or drug-drug interactions are also multiplied.[3] Drug-taking behavior of the elderly may be an additional source of difficulty, owing to the increased prevalence of confusion or outright dementia in many elderly patients, as well as the heightened complexity of their regimens. Finally, it is important not to lose sight of the socioeconomic aspects of drug utilization in this age group. With pharmaceutical products comprising one of the highest out-of-pocket health care expenses for those over 65, the economic impact of drug utilization or misutilization is particularly important for this group of patients who often live on fixed and barely adequate incomes.[4]

For all of these reasons, one would have good reason to expect a much higher frequency of adverse drug reactions in the elderly, as compared with younger groups. This is not meant to underestimate the very positive effects that medications in general have on the elderly population, many of whose

This work was supported by grants from the National Center for Health Services Research, National Institute on Aging, and the AARP-Andrus Foundation.

members benefit greatly from the therapies that we have to offer them. Nonetheless, the focus of the present discussion is the negative consequences of drugs in this age group, and this is an area to which further attention will need to be paid as the population becomes an increasingly elderly one in this country as well as in most of the industrialized world. Given the increasing interest in how we are to pay for the health care of the elderly, study of their drug utilization also carries with it important economic and policy considerations, as well as the obvious clinical and epidemiologic questions.

For the last several years, members of the Harvard Medical School drug epidemiology unit have been studying several aspects of the utilization of drugs in the population in general, and in the aged in particular. In this work, we have increasingly been drawn to the potential usefulness of data from the Medicaid programs of several states as a repository of useful data concerning several of the issues in which we have been interested. This chapter will present reports of our work in two areas that have made use of such data: drug utilization patterns, with particular reference to inappropriate prescribing by physicians; and postmarketing surveillance of drugs for adverse effects in the elderly.

Our work on defining and reducing inappropriate prescribing by physicians has been based on the premise that important facts about the indications, efficacy, and inefficacy of various drugs are often not brought to physicians' attention as forcefully as are facts about newer agents, still under patent and therefore promoted vigorously by their manufacturers. As a result, it is often difficult for physicians to keep perspective on the very rapidly changing field of pharmacology, and numerous instances can be cited in which prescribing is less than optimal. It has been argued that medical schools have abrogated their responsibility in this area and could take a much stronger role in actually reaching out to physicians to provide them with the latest information on drug choices unaffected by commercial considerations, which of necessity play a large role in the promotional activities of the industry.[5]

Our hypothesis was simple: It should be possible to improve the accuracy of physician prescribing behavior, and contain costs as well, if a medical school adopted the same sophisticated (and often elegant) methods of communication employed by the private sector, but with the communication aimed at reducing inappropriate prescribing rather than promoting sales of a particular product.[6,7] Because self-reporting by physicians is a very poor way of knowing exactly what is being prescribed, we obtained data from four state Medicaid programs with sophisticated Medicaid Management Information Systems (MMIS) to study patterns of drug utilization supported through their programs. Four hundred and thirty-five physicians were identified who were moderate to high prescribers of three drug groups we selected for our educational program; propoxyphene (eg, Darvon and others), the cerebral and peripheral "vasodilators" promoted for the treatment of senility and claudication, and cephalexin (eg, Keflex), a cephalosporin antibiotic. The rationale was that propoxyphene is increasingly considered not to be an analgesic of choice, and considerable evidence indicates that it has little to recommend it over aspirin or acetaminophen; there is virtual unanimity among geriatricians that the so-called cerebral and peripheral vasodilators are of essentially no use in the treatment of either senile dementia or peripheral and vascular insufficiency. The third drug, cephalexin, is, unlike the other two, quite effective but is probably over-utilized to a considerable degree as it is widely prescribed for outpatient problems for which a much cheaper, older antibiotic, or no antibiotic at all, would be the most appropriate therapy.

The physicians in our sample were randomized into three groups. The control group received no intervention whatever; the "print-only" group received a series of mailed "un-advertisements" as well as a number of materials directed specifically at patients concerning the drugs in question (see Figures 12.1 and 12.2). The "face-to-face" group received these printed materials as well as visits by a team of drug educators, clinical pharmacists by training, whom we provided with additional training in both the pharmacology of the drugs in question and techniques of communication and behavior change.

The results of the experiment were clear-cut, and generally bore out our hypothesis. Physicians randomized into the face-to-face group decreased their prescribing of the target drugs significantly ($P=.003$) when compared with control physicians. Some small change was also seen in the expected direction in the print-only group, but it did not reach statistical significance (Figures 12.3, 12.4).

Receptivity on the part of physicians visited by our drug information specialists was very high, with 92% agreeing to participate in the educational visits, most of them quite enthusiastically.[8] (For purposes of data analysis, all physicians randomized into the face-to-face group, whether they participated in the intervention or not, were considered as one group.) In an attempt to measure the economic consequences of our program, we were careful to measure (using the same Medicaid prescribing data base) physicians' utilization of potential substitute drugs, which may have undercut the reductions we observed in their prescribing of the target drugs. Every conceivable substitution was analyzed, and the only one that came even close to appearing significant was an increase in the use of over-the-counter analgesics such as aspirin or acetaminophen instead of propoxyphene, which we had encouraged. Even this effect was a slight one, but to be conservative the economic consequences of this change were analyzed in performing our analysis. In brief, we found that the amount of money saved by the Medicaid programs of the four participating states was *greater* than the amount that it would cost to continue such a program on an operational basis. The formal benefit-cost analysis that we have performed bears out this conclusion in great detail, and serves as an interesting foundation for future consideration of the policy relevance of this approach.[9] It is not often that one can

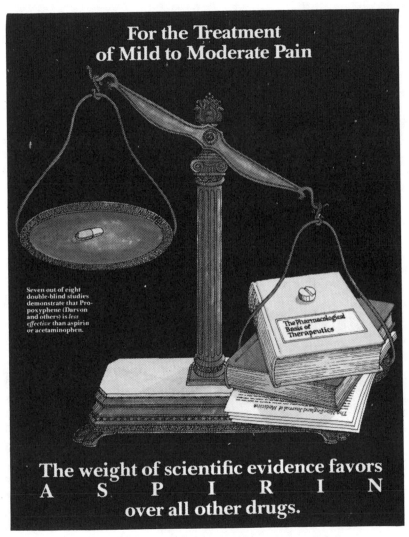

Figure 12.1. Example of "unadvertisement" used in
the prescribing interventions described in the text.

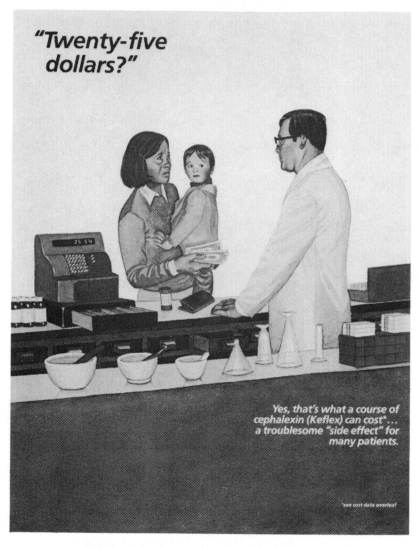

Figure 12.2. Example of "unadvertisement" used
in the prescribing interventions   described in the text.

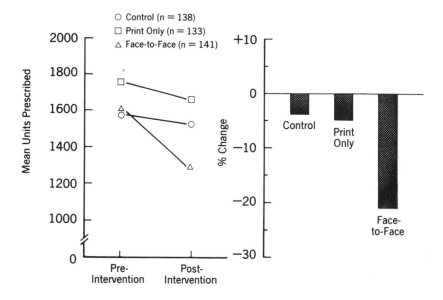

Figure 12.3. Reduction in prescribing of all target drugs as a result of the intervention described in the text. The face-to-face group result differed from that of controls at a significance level of $p=.003$; the print group did not differ signicantly from the control.

document, in a randomized controlled trial, a health care intervention that both improves patient care and reduces costs at the same time. Such an approach would seem particularly appropriate for any health service delivery organization that finds itself footing the bill for drug expenditures of its patients, such as health maintenance organizations, the Veterans Administration, the various state Medicaid programs, and certain national health service programs abroad.[10] Discussions are underway with several groups of this nature concerning implementation of this approach on a wider scale.

Our work in the epidemiology of adverse drug reactions in the elderly is in a much earlier stage of development. The essence of the approach is to take hypotheses generated at the clinical level that relate to possible adverse drug effects in the aged and test them by means of the same kind of computerized analysis of Medicaid data. Thus far, much of this work has been done on the Computerized On-Line Pharmaceutical Analysis and Surveillance System (COMPASS) system developed by Health Information Designs (HID) for the Food and Drug Administration. As in the prescribing research just described, this approach makes use of the wealth of data contained in the MMIS files that has thus far been used by the states primarily for reimbursement purposes.[11,12] Tapes containing enormous amounts of data on a claim-by-claim basis, generally in no particular order, are shipped to HID

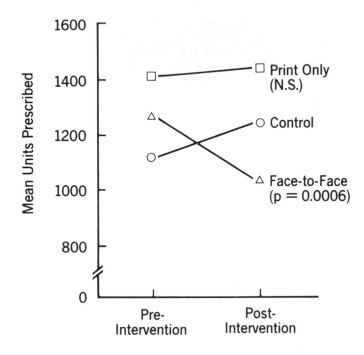

Figure 12.4. Changes in prescribing of the costly antibiotic cephalexin by physicians before and after the Harvard study. Triangles represent physicians randomized into the "un-detail" group; their prescribing of cephalexin dropped while that of physicians in the control group (circles) was on the increase. Physicians who received only mailed "un-advertisements" did not change prescribing significantly.

where they are sorted and put into a format that makes them epidemiologically accessible. Claims for all prescriptions filled, all ambulatory visits to physicians, hospitalizations, and nursing home stays are sorted into files by recipient identification number, drug name (in the NDC format), and diagnosis (in the ICD-9-CM format). These are arranged in a temporal sequence, so that it becomes possible to retrieve a profile of all health-related encounters experienced by a given Medicaid recipient for a period that now runs from the beginning of 1980 through the end of 1983 and is being updated continuously. Nearly 2 million Medicaid recipients are included in the "core" COMPASS data base, with several million more from other states being added to the system presently.

Like any secondary data set, there are limitations to this approach that must be taken into account in any research. Data relating to drug utilization are probably the most valid in the system, owing to the nonambiguity of the way in which prescriptions are recorded and the necessity of correct and complete recording before reimbursement is made to the pharmacist.[13,14] It appears that principal hospital diagnoses are also of fairly good validity for research purposes. We look with a more jaundiced eye upon diagnoses based on physician office visits, because these may represent only one of several ongoing illnesses, particularly in this population, and we reserve the greatest skepticism for nursing home diagnoses, since these records, like much else in the typical nursing home medical record, may bear only slight resemblance to the actual health status of the patient. Because of the particularly high validity of the drug data base in this system, we have been exploring ways in which the prescription of certain medications can be used as a "marker" for the presence of a particular illness (eg, antidepressants for depression, bladder-active agents for incontinence, and so forth).

Considerable promise exists in the potential use of such enormous computer-based data sets for research into the epidemiology of drug effects, as well as health services utilization in the elderly. Our group is currently studying a number of geriatric-type outcomes in relation to medication use as well as utilization of other health services, such as nursing home care. The conditions under most active scrutiny in our unit currently include falls and fractures, urinary incontinence, hypertension, and depression. Subsequent reports will provide details of our findings in each of these areas.

In summary, we believe that a number of factors have come together in the last few years to make possible an important new approach to the study of drug utilization and drug epidemiology. First is the refinement of data that are routinely collected as part of the management systems of several very large health care systems, such as Medicaid and Medicare.[15,16] It should be noted that the accuracy of diagnoses in these categories will probably be affected greatly as the diagnosis-related group (DRG) approach to reimbursement becomes ever more universal. A second development of importance is the escalating sophistication of the computer software and hardware necessary to manipulate such enormous data bases, which were, until recently, too unwieldy for any but the biggest main-frame computer applications. Third is the increasing awareness of the need to better define the outcomes of drug utilization in this highly vulnerable group of elderly, spurred on in part by an increasing awareness by both clinicians and the public alike of the potential disasters that await us if we are not vigilant in this area. Fourth is the development, which is only about a decade old, of geriatrics as a field of expertise within medicine, with its own particular set of research questions — questions which have for too long been neglected by the rest of the medical community.

Given the intersection of these various trends in the last ten years, the stage is now set for some very exciting new work on drug utilization, with particular reference to the group that consumes medications in the highest quantity and is in greatest need of creative research concerning their effects.

REFERENCES

1. Avorn J, Lamy P, Vestal R: Prescribing for the elderly. *Patient Care* 1982; 16(12):14–62.

2. Greenblatt DJ, Sellers EM, Shader RI: Drug therapy: Drug disposition in old age. *N Engl J Med* 1982; 306:1081–1088.

3. Conrad KA, Bressler R (eds): *Drug Therapy for the Elderly.* St Louis, CV Mosby Co, 1982.

4. Avorn J: Drug policy in the aging society. *Health Affairs* 1983; 2:23–32.

5. Rucker TD: Drug information for prescribers and dispensers: Toward a model system. *Med Care* 1976; 14:156–165.

6. Avorn J, Chen M, Hartley R: Scientific vs commercial sources of influence on physician prescribing behavior. *Am J Med* 1982; 73:4-8

7. Temin P: *Taking Your Medicine: Drug Regulation in the United States.* Cambridge, MA, Harvard University Press, 1980.

8. Avorn J, Soumerai SB: Improving drug-therapy decisions through educational outreach: A randomized controlled trial of academically based "detailing." *N Engl J Med* 1983; 308:1457–1463.

9. Soumerai SB, Avorn J: Medical school drug education outreach: A cost-effective approach to quality assurance (submitted for publication).

10. Avorn J: Containing the cost of improper prescribing. *Business and Health* 1984; 1(4): 35–39.

11. LeRoy AA, Morse ML: *An Evaluation of the Use of Title XIX Medicaid Management Information System as a Data Resource for Conducting Post-Marketing Drug Surveillance Studies. Report to the Bureau of Drugs, Food and Drug Administration.* Washington, DC, 1980.

12. Office of Technology Assessment, U.S. Congress: *Post-Marketing Surveillance of Prescription Drugs.* Washington, DC, 1982.

13. Ray WA, Federspiel CF, Schaffner W: A study of antipsychotic drug use in nursing homes: Epidemiologic evidence suggesting misuse. *Am J Public Health* 1980; 70:485–491.

14. Blazer DG, Federspiel CF, Ray WA, et al: The risk of anticholinergic toxicity in the elderly: A study of prescribing practices in two populations. *J Gerontol* 1983; 38(1):31–36.

15. Roos LL, Nicol JP, Johnson CF, et al: Using administrative data banks for research and evaluation: A case study. *Eval Quarterly* 1979; 3(2):236–255.

16. Federspiel CF, Ray WA, Schaffner W: Medicaid records as a valid data source: The Tennessee experience. *Med Care* 1976; 14(2):166–172.

Chapter 13

POSTMARKETING SURVEILLANCE (PMS) AND GERIATRIC DRUG USE

Fred Wegner

The concept of a comprehensive national system of postmarketing surveillance (PMS) is the Harold Stassen of drug politics and policy. Recommendations for a national system of PMS emerge with just about the same quadrennial frequency as Harold Stassen's announcements of presidential availability. And they go back about as far.

The first mention I came across was in 1966 when D.J. Finney in *Proceedings of the European Society for the Study of Drug Toxicity* stated that "... the monitoring of adverse reactions must become part of the regular framework of health services. . . . It is a response to a need to replace haphazard collection and interpretation of information by something more organized. . . ."

That was 18 years ago. Four years later, in 1970, the report of the International Conference on Adverse Reactions Reporting Systems set forth the need for a national approach to drug surveillance.

Four years after that, a PMS recommendation again surfaced, this time in a published paper by Medicine in the Public Interest, which is an organization funded by some drug manufacturers.

In 1980, Harold Stassen's hat was in the ring again, and the final report of the Joint Commission on Prescription Drug Use concluded that a national Center for Drug Surveillance was necessary to coordinate and build on already existing PMS functions.

Now it's 4 years later. Stassen has reemerged and so has discussion of a comprehensive national system of postmarketing surveillance.

To complete the ill-starred history of PMS to date, I should mention the joint effort of the FDA and the Experimental Technology Incentives Program (ETIP) of the National Bureau of Standards. The project, entitled "An Experiment in Early Post-Marketing Surveillance of Drugs," was contracted to IMS American and carried out between January 1978 and September 1980.

The Task A report — 337 pages — described existing methods of post-marketing surveillance and evaluated their strengths and limitations. The Task B report — 393 pages — identified feasible and potentially useful methods of PMS, and the Task C report — 371 pages — was a visualization of a comprehensive national postmarketing surveillance system and recommendations for the methodologic elements needed for its operation.

In a 1980 article about this project, Jerry Halperin wrote about the enthusiasm, the high expectations, the fact that it was "highly visible around the world." Four years later, so far as I know, all 1,101 pages of "An Experiment in Early Post-Marketing Surveillance of Drugs" lie smoldering in the grave of the National Technical Information Service in Springfield, Virginia.

What is meant by a comprehensive national PMS system? Here we find differences of opinion as to priorities and emphasis. The FDA-ETIP study listed the concerns of PMS as these:

• Discovery of adverse effects unsuspected at the time of marketing

• Quantification of suspected or known adverse effects

• Quantification of efficacy and the discovery of new indications

To these basic needs, other observers have added further clarifications and requirements: Together with the need to quantify adverse drug reactions (ADRs) is the need to be more specific about the findings. We need to know more not only about the severity of the ADRs, but about the severity of the treated illness. Similarly, we need to know more about the exact nature of patient noncompliance and medication errors — not only rates, but types.

We need to know the effects on special populations — especially those not included or underrepresented in Phase III studies — such as the elderly and children, pregnant women, patients with diseases other than the one being studied, patients taking other medications, as well as the increased risk of effects due to other factors such as lifestyle, smoking, and so on. And we need long-term and follow-up studies that will cover the effects of drugs in the fetus and effects that manifest only after long use or delays.

Is this a tall order? I don't think so; especially in this country at this time. I often feel the United States resembles nothing so much as a giant data bank: we have figures and models on virtually everything. What could be improved upon are priorities. A lot more is known about baseball players and games than about patients and drugs. There is no dearth of ad hoc and partial PMS studies in the literature both here and abroad. Neither is there a lack of recommendations and analyses of a comprehensive national PMS system. What we have yet to see is a serious legislative or regulatory proposal to implement a national PMS system.

It is disappointing in most of what we hear and read about a formal PMS system that so little attention is devoted to the educational and informational aspects. After all these data are obtained, what then? The logical and paramount consequence is to improve health and to do that by improving prescribing practices, by increasing patients' knowledge so as to improve their behavior in drug therapy, and by averting such factors that cause ADRs.

All of these goals are important and beneficial, and they will not be realized to their fullest by the limited means of simply changing the professional labeling of the drug. We know that many doctors prescribe outside the constraints of the official labeling. And without official, comprehensive, and universal patient labeling, polls show us that one of the greatest unfulfilled consumer needs today is for patient drug information.

It may be far easier and of greater interest to the editors of medical journals to deal with PMS systems and data-gathering, but these pursuits in and of themselves will not improve health, prescribing, compliance, or behavior.

While we are waiting — perhaps another 4 years — for a national PMS system, it would be useful to see advances in the state of the art of patient information and education.

PART 6

RESEARCH IN
ELDERLY DRUG RESPONSES

Chapter 14

SURVEY OF DRUG USE AND MENTAL DISORDERS IN NURSING HOMES

Mary S. Harper, RN, PhD

OVERVIEW OF AGING IN THE UNITED STATES

In the United States, there are 24.4 million persons over 65 years of age. Five thousand individuals become 65 years of age daily. Today, one out of every five Americans is 60 or older. In the next 55 years, the population will increase by 35%: The over 65 population group will increase 119% and the over 85 population will increase even more, by 206%. The rate of increase is greater for the black elderly than it is for the white elderly. Between 1970 and 1980, older black Americans experienced a 34% increase as compared with a 23% increase for the white elderly. There are many implications for policy formulation, manpower development, and allocation of health, social, and economic resources.[1,2]

In the United States, we are challenged in providing for the 24.4 million people over 64 years old. Our national government's existing policy commitments toward the elderly currently lead it to spend one-fourth of the annual federal budget on programs for the aging ($132.2 billion out of a total $531.6 billion in fiscal year 1980), a constituency of 24.4 million persons aged 65 and older who comprise 11% of our population. The present policies do not

The author would like to express her appreciation to Dr John Bell, Executive Director, Mrs Julia Trocchio, and Mrs Kathy O'Donoghue of the American Health Care Association for collaboration in this survey. I wish to acknowledge with appreciation the assistance provided by Dr Ronald Manderscheid and Dr Barabara Burns of NIMH Biometry Division and Dr Barry Lebowitz, Chief of the Center for Studies of the Mental Health of the Aging, in the development of the questionnaire and the sampling design.

substantially alleviate the severest problems of poverty, ill health, substandard housing, and inadequate social services experienced by millions of the most disadvantaged elderly.[3]

If the present policies are maintained, the mere demographic increase in the number and proportion of older persons in the United States will lead annual federal expenditures on aging to more than triple in real dollars early in the next century and to constitute 40% of total federal outlays. Each year the fiscal, humanitarian, and political problems involved in this dilemma are exacerbated and the options for resolving them become more limited.[3,4] The figures here represent those of the federal government; they do not include the state and local expenditures for aging programs. It is a challenge for survival to the federal as well as the state and local governments.

Actually, most of the elderly are active and in relatively good health until the age of 75 or 80. We must not generalize about the elderly. Bernice Neugarten[5] has categorized the young-old as aged 55 to 75 and the old-old as 75+. It is useful for policymakers, health planners, administrators, and others to use this categorization in analysis of the aging data. For example, most elderly people are capable of carrying out all of the activities of daily living until the age of 80; therefore, special health policies and entitlements are generally needed for those 80+ years of age and not those 55 to 75 years of age.

NURSING HOMES IN THE UNITED STATES

There are 23,065 nursing homes in the United States. Of the 23,065, 19,900 are certified. There are 1.5 million beds with 1.4 million persons in nursing homes. There are more persons in nursing homes than are in all of the acute hospitals. Nursing homes are the fastest growing health industry.[6] In 1981, the national health expenditures for nursing homes were $24 billion. The U.S. Department of Health and Human Services nursing home expenditures will quadruple by 1990, reaching $81.9 billion. Nursing home residents generally suffer multiple conditions, and two thirds of them have two to three chronic diseases.

BEHAVIORAL, SOCIAL, EMOTIONAL, AND MENTAL DISORDERS IN THE NURSING HOME

Various surveys and studies have reported that 46% to 75% of the residents in nursing homes have behavioral, social, emotional, and mental disorders.[7-10]

Many of the nation's nursing homes are rapidly becoming major institutions for long-term care of the mentally ill.[10,11] In addition, they house a sizable population of individuals now having or at risk of having mental, behavioral, or emotional problems. Several studies have reported that current resources of nursing homes appear to be inadequate to respond to the mental health needs of their residents — whether in the realm of prevention, treatment, rehabilitation, or training of their staff in psychogerontology or psychogeriatrics. There is a lack of systematic approach to the care of persons with behavioral, social, and emotional problems, as well as to the mentally ill in nursing homes.[6-8]

The elderly suffer disproportionately from psychiatric disorders. Organic brain disease increases after age 60 and the suicide rate is highest in elderly white males. Two National Institute of Mental Health (NIMH) studies[12,13] listed the following incidence of new cases of psychopathology of all types per 100,000 population: age 25 to 34 — 76.3; age 35 to 64 — 93.0; and above age 65 — 236.1. The incidence of functional disorders — notably depression and paranoid states — increases with age.[14] Other studies have found a 30% prevalence of diagnosable psychiatric disorders in the over 65 population, with about 15% likely to be severely disabled.[15,16] Depression accounts for about half of all psychiatric disorders in the elderly. Busse and Wang[17] found support that brief episodes of depression afflict 25% of normal people over 60. They stress that the commonest precipitant is decline in physical health. Felix Post[18] believes that in many people with lifelong neurotic symptoms, depressive illness with largely neurotic symptomatology develops in later life. Physiological, psychological, and psychosocial precipitants are of greater significance in depression first occurring in people over 50 than they are in younger depressives. Losses, symbolic or concrete, are the most common factors.

Symptoms such as fatigue, apathy, insomnia, headache, abdominal pain, pain all over, anorexia, constipation, incontinence, urinary urgency, diarrhea, "passing out," confusion, and diffuse pains represent a wide range of human reactivity to psychological disorders as well as physical illness; a myriad of psychiatric symptoms ranging from apathy to manic depression have been associated with specific medical and psychiatric diseases. Several studies have shown a close relationship between physical symptoms and psychopathology in the elderly. Pfeiffer and Busse noted that 33% of the elderly in any community have an anxious preoccupation with bodily functions. Salzman found 64% of elderly individuals hospitalized for depression to have "physically unjustified bodily complaints," most frequently involving the gastrointestinal tract, the head, or the cardiovascular system.[9]

USE OF DRUGS BY THE ELDERLY IN NURSING HOMES

Studies show that multiple drug therapy or polypharmacy is a common practice worldwide.[19-21] Many agencies and countries find themselves faced with the trend toward overuse of drugs in general by the elderly population. In view of the very high proportion of total drug consumption accounted for by the elderly (perhaps in excess of 50%) the World Health Organization (WHO) feels that the problem urgently needs to be dealt with.[19]

In the United States of America, the elderly represent 11.4% of the population and consume one-third of the 1.5 billion prescriptions written each year. By the year 2000, the elderly will consume 50% of all the prescriptions written. The over-65 population uses an average of 14 prescriptions per year, which is nearly twice the average amount used by persons between the ages of 25 and 54. Approximately two thirds of all older persons use nonprescription drugs on a regular basis.[22] The drug industry is a $25 billion industry: the fourth largest health care expenditure.

The elderly are great consumers of drugs; therefore, they have a high percentage of the adverse drug effects/reactions as well as drug-related iatrogenic disease.[22-24]

Levenson et al[23] found the following rates of iatrogenic disease in various age groups: a 21.3% rate of iatrogenic disease in the 70 to 79 age group as compared to a 3% rate in the 20 to 29 age group. Another survey (performed by Levenson and cited in Levenson et al[23]) revealed a 24.9% rate of iatrogenic disease in the 80+ age group versus a 9.9% rate in the 21 to 30 age group.

Twelve to 18% of the admissions (300,000) are the result of drug reactions, which cost $3 billion each year, and 30,000 people who are under professional supervision die each year from adverse drug reactions.[22]

The most frequently used groups of drugs in nursing homes include: diuretics, antidepressives, tranquilizers and psychomimetics, digitalis, hypnotic sedatives/anticonvulsants, analgesics and antipyretics, hypotensives, and tremor and rigidity controllers.[21, 22, 25-27]

It has been found that the elderly are heavy consumers of the drugs with the highest degrees of risk producing more adverse drug reactions. There is a paucity of information on the pharmacokinetics and pharmacodynamics of drugs used most frequently by the elderly. The elderly are generally excluded from clinical trials. Information is available on younger persons, whereas in the elderly we must rely on trial and error, clinical impressions, and anecdotal data.

Reindenberg[28] has summarized a group of research studies concerning drugs and the elderly patient indicating that (1) digitalis toxicity is a more common occurrence in the older patient, primarily due to renal function, (2) drug metabolism is generally slower in elderly patients, (3) a considerably higher percentage of patients over 65 admitted to psychiatric services require hospitalization as a direct result of psychotropic drug effects.[27]

PSYCHOTROPIC DRUGS AND THE ELDERLY IN THE NURSING HOME

From 1973 to 1974, of 1,075,800 nursing home residents, 96% received at least one type of medication: tranquilizers, hypnotic-sedatives, stool softeners, antidepressants, diuretics, analgesics, diabetic agents, antihypertensives, cardiac glycosides, antiinflammatory agents, antiinfectives, antianginal drugs, anticoagulants, and vitamins and iron in the week prior to data collection.[29]

Nearly half (48%, or 482,600) of those taking medications received tranquilizers, and 38% received vitamin or iron supplements. The report states that the number receiving tranquilizers may be underestimated. The number of residents taking medication was 890,000. Over 8% (8.9%, or 91,300) of the residents received antidepressants and 34.4% (or 355,200) received hypnotic-sedatives. The profile for residents receiving tranquilizers and hypnotic-sedatives and antidepressants in the 1977 nursing home survey[29] was similar to the directions listed above. In the 1977 survey, 36% of the residents received tranquilizers. A larger proportion of the residents who were mentally ill (69%) or mentally retarded (65%) received tranquilizers than did the residents with other conditions. However, the use of tranquilizers by all residents in nursing homes is high; in a study of 283,915 residents in a skilled nursing facility (SNF), it was found that 1,731,360 prescriptions were written (average of 6.1 per resident) with a range of 0 to 23 per resident — 51.3% of the prescriptions were written for tranquilizers.[25]

It has been well established by other studies that there is a high percentage of persons in nursing homes with emotional, social, behavioral, and mental disorders who are receiving one or more psychotropic drugs. It is of interest that many of the recipients of psychotropic drugs do not have a psychiatric diagnosis.[23-25, 30]

In 1968, the HEW task force on prescription drugs[31] reported that the three most commonly prescribed drugs for the elderly were diazepam, chlordiazepoxide, and the nonnarcotic analgesic propoxyphene. In another survey[32] of a long-term care facility, psychotropic drugs were shown to be the most commonly prescribed (61%), followed by diuretics and antihypertensive drugs (46%), and antimicrobials (14%) and cardiotonics (15%).[20]

PRESENT STUDY

Little is known about the emotional, social, behavioral, and mental disorders of the individual residents in nursing homes. Neither is much known about the mental health manpower; treatment resources in the institution and community; barriers to use of psychiatric treatment resources and manpower (ie, how frequently do nursing homes use community mental health centers [CMHC], state hospitals, psychiatrists, psychatric nurses, social workers and psychologists for consultation); what drugs or combination of drugs are used for what kinds of behaviors, conditions, and diagnoses; what is a fairly *authentic working profile of the diagnoses* of residents with emotional, behavioral, and mental disorders — not the reimbursable diagnosis.

Such information would assist the association and agency to plan and evaluate programmatic directions and identify needs and barriers to research and manpower development. Our questionnaire was developed in two parts. Part I included such demographic items as:

I.   Description of facility, classification as to skilled nursing facility (SNF) or intermediate care facility (ICF), the number of certified Medicare/Medicaid beds

II.   Description of resident population

    A. Number of male and female residents

    B. Percentage of residents by age (ie, 61 to 70, 71 to 80, 81 to 90, and 91 to 100)

III.   Admission and discharge

    A. Their homes

    B. Another nursing home

    C. Acute CRE hospital

    D. State mental hospital

    E. Boarding home/domiciliary

    F. VA medical center

    G. Other

IV.   Diagnosis

    A. What percentage of residents have primary psychiatric diagnosis? (ie, up to 10%, 11% to 20%, 21% to 30%, 31% to 40%, etc)

    B. What percentage of residents have a secondary psychiatric diagnosis and *not* a primary psychiatric diagnosis?

    C. What percentage of residents display mental, emotional psychological, or social behavioral problems?

V.   Services: psychiatric case consultation is provided by frequency of the services; frequently, seldom, don't know, and on call

    A. Psychiatrist

    B. Psychologist

    C. Psychiatric nurse, psychiatric social worker

    D. State mental hospital

E. Community mental health center (CMHC)

F. None of the above

G. Other

VI. Full-time, part-time, and consulting staff

VII. Are the CMHC's resources utilized by nursing home residents or staff?

A. If yes, what type of services are used?

B. If no, what are the barriers to use of CMHC's resources by the nursing homes?

VIII. When residents have behavioral or mental disorders interfering with their physical, social, and interpersonal functioning and relationships, which of the following actions do you generally take?

	Frequent	Seldom	Usual	Never
Transfer to state hospital	___	___	___	___
Transfer to a special security room	___	___	___	___
Put in restraints	___	___	___	___
Lock in a room to prevent injury to self and others	___	___	___	___
Call a psychologist/mental health psychiatric nurse for consultation	___	___	___	___
Ask the physician to order psychotropic drugs	___	___	___	___
Request consultation from the nearest community mental health center	___	___	___	___

IX. Do you have an overall policy or regulation that prohibits admission of residents with a psychiatric diagnosis or disturbed behaviors?

X. Do you have a closed unit for psychiatric patients or persons with behavioral disorders?

XI. How many hours of organized instruction and supervised practice do you have for the following employees?

_____ Nurses' aides

_____ Food service workers

_____ Licensed Practical Nurses

XII.   Do you have orientation for each of the following? If so, please check
       the appropriate space for how many hours:

                                              Number of Hours
                                           5   10   20   None

       Physicians
       Psychologists
       Social workers
       Registered Nurses
       Licensed Practical Nurses
       Nurses' aides
       Food servers

Part II of the questionnaire was for the individual resident. One form was
completed for each of the 10 residents with a primary or secondary psychiatric
diagnosis or behavioral problems. There were 50 items relating to diagnosis
and behavior; 15 items relating to therapy and the use of clinical staff (physical therapist, podiatrist, dentist, speech therapist, psychotherapist, etc); 63
items relating to drugs (most were psychotropic, antidepressants, hypnotic
sedatives, etc).

SAMPLING DESIGN

Initially, 600 nursing homes were randomly selected from the 1,800 mem-
bership list of the American Health Care Association Computer. Two
hundred nursing homes were then selected for study (see Table 14.1).

Table 14.1. Data from Nursing Home Study

Size of Nursing Homes	Number of Residents From Each Size Home	Number of Nursing Homes in This Category	Percentage of The Sample
Large (100 plus beds)	15	120	60
Intermediary (70 plus beds)	10	60	30
Small (40 plus beds)	5	20	10
	2,500 residents	200 nursing homes	100

We anticipated specific data on 2,500 residents from 200 nursing homes
categorized as large, intermediate and small.

Two hundred forty-three questionnaires were returned from 30 nursing
homes. A follow-up letter will be sent out in mid-1984.

Approximately 7% (6.7%) of the nursing homes responded, returning 10%
of the questionnaires.

Some of the findings from the first 100 questionnaires returned included:

1. Fifty percent of the residents had two to three diagnoses (ie, senile dementia, mental retardation, and anxiety disorders).

2. Most frequently reported diagnosis included:
   A. Mental retardation (15)
   B. Organic brain syndrome (27)
   C. Senile dementia (25)
   D. Depressive disorder (25)
   E. Schizophrenia (15)
   F. Anxiety disorder (20)
   G. Personality/character disorder (30)

3. The most common behaviors described included:
   A. Confusion (75)
   B. Oriented as to time (21)
   C. Oriented as to place (35)
   D. Oriented as to person (40)
   E. Depressed (70)
   F. Feelings of unworthiness (60)
   G. Trouble concentrating (54)
   H. Irritable (impatient and easily annoyed and restless) (68)
   I. Easily distracted (72)

4. More questionnaires (40%) were returned from large intermediate care facilities (ICF) than from skilled nursing facilities (SNF). The SNF returning questionnaires were small.

5. More questionnaires were returned on the female residents. The highest percentage of the residents were in the 81 to 90 age bracket.

6. An even number of residents were admitted from acute care hospitals, other nursing homes, state mental hospitals.

7. Twenty percent of the residents had a primary psychiatric diagnosis.

8. Forty-five percent of the residents had a secondary psychiatric diagnosis.

9. Eighty percent of the residents displayed mental, emotional, psychological, or behavioral problems.

10. Consultation was most frequently provided by the psychiatric nurse, next by the psychiatrist, and third by the social worker; none of the nursing homes had a full-time psychiatrist. Only one nursing home used a psychologist as a consultant. Only 30% of the nursing homes had

a full-time physician there with no psychiatrist on call. Several of the respondents stated that the barrier to using the CMHC was that their staff was not trained to work with the elderly.

11. When a resident displayed disturbed behavior, the three most frequent courses of action were: Request the physician to order a psychotropic drug, request consultation from the nearby CMHC, and transfer the patient to state hospital. Placing the resident in seclusion and restraints was seldom used.

12. Only one nursing home had a policy that prohibited admission of a person with a psychiatric diagnosis or disturbed behavior.

13. Only one nursing home had a "closed" or special unit for residents with a psychiatric diagnosis or disturbed behavior.

14. All of the nursing homes had in-service education programs or orientation for nurses, licensed practical nurses, or nursing aides; none of them had orientation/in-service for psychologists; and one had orientation for physicians.

15. Most frequently used drugs included:

A. Chlorpromazine HCl (Thorazine) (20) generally given b.i.d.

B. Thioridazine (Mellaril) (14) generally given t.i.d.

C. Phenobarbital (11) generally given t.i.d.

D. Benadryl (8) generally given daily

E. Haloperidol (Haldol) (25) generally given daily

F. Thiothixene (Navane) (10) generally given daily
G. Flurazepam HCl (Dalmane) (7) generally given daily

H. Chloral hydrate (5) generally given daily
I. Chlordiazepoxide HCl (Librium) (3) generally given B.I.D.

J. Fluphenazine (Prolixin decanoate) (3) generally given daily

K. Amitriptyline HCl (Elavil) (4) generally given daily

L. Lithium carbonate (1) generally given t.i.d.

M. Doxepin HCl (Sinequan) (3)

N. Imipramine HCl (Tofranil) (3)

O. Triavil (3)

P. Mesoridazine (Serentil) (3) generally given daily

Q. Benztropine mesylate (Cogentin) generally given t.i.d.

R. Artane (3) generally given t.i.d.

S. Lorazepam (Ativan) (2) generally given b.i.d.

T. Loxapine succinate (Loxitane) (3) generally given t.i.d.

U. Ludiomil (3) generally given t.i.d.

V. Beer or wine (3) generally given t.i.d. and h.s.

From the preceding report, there is evidence that the elderly are heavy users of psychotropic drugs, although little is known about the pharmodynamics and the pharmacokinetics of these drugs in the elderly. Adverse drug reactions occur seven times more often in the elderly than they do in persons 20 to 29 years of age.

With most of the elderly on multiple drugs, one must be cautioned of drug-drug interactions as well as drug-food interactions that could produce exaggerated pharmacologic reactions. This can occur at the site of drug action, or it may affect the absorption, distribution, metabolism, or excretion of the drugs. Recent studies reviewing drug literature and profiles of nursing home patients showed the potential for significant reactions in 53% of drugs administered.[27, 33]

For the most part, psychotropic drugs are detoxified by the liver.[34] The liver does demonstrate substantial age-related changes. The number of hepatocytes decreases markedly with increasing age as represented by liver mass. There is generally a change of 25% to 30% decrease in liver mass in patients aged 60 years as compared to those 40 years of age. Additionally, Zaske[35] reports that various enzymatic pathways of drug detoxification also demonstrate decreased activity. Drugs that commonly induce these enzymes in younger patients, such as phenobarbital, do not have the same propensity in elderly persons compared to those 40 years of age and directly decrease liver blood flow. Consequently, drugs such as the psychotropics metabolized by the liver demonstrate a decreased effectiveness in the aged.

Therefore, more research is needed as to pharmacokinetics and pharmodynamics of psychotropic drugs and the elderly now that the high prevalence of mental disorders and the high use of psychotropic drugs for nursing home residents have been established. However, it must be remembered that the elderly are a very heterogeneous group.

REFERENCES

1. Rabushka A: Aging and public policy: Rethinking issues and programs. *Grants Magazine* 1980; 3(3):152-156.

2. Reid J: *Black Americans in the 1980s — Population Bulletin.* Washington, DC, Population Reference Bureau, Inc (Vol. 37, No. 4) 1982.

3. Binstock RH: Introductory overview, in Binstock RH, Chow W-S, Schylz XX: *International Perspectives on Aging: Population and Policy Challenges.* New York, United Nations Fund for Population Activities, Policy Development Studies (No. 7, PPT-VIII).

4. Kutza EA: The impact of federal programs on older persons. *National Forum* 1982; 13(4):6-8.

5. Neugarten BL: The future and the young-old. *Gerontologist* 1951; SV(1):4-9.

6. Kane RL, Kane RA: Care of the aged: Old problems in need of new solutions. *Science* 1978; 200:913-918.

7. U.S. National Center for Health Statistics: *National Health Survey (Series 13, No. 27)* Washington, DC U.S. Government Printing Office, 1977.

8. Cohen G: Mental health services and the elderly: Needs and options. *American Journal of Psychiatry* 1976; 65-68.

9. Ouslander JG: Illness and psychopathology in the elderly. *Psych Clin North Am.*

10. Department of Health and Human Services: *Toward a National Plan for the Chronically Mentally Ill* (Steering Committee on the Chronically Mentally Ill Report). Washington, DC, DHHS, 1981. DHHS Publication No. (ADM) 81-1077.

11. Department of Health and Human Services: *Care of the Mentally Ill in Nursing Homes. (Addendum Toward a National Plan for the Chronically Mentally Ill)* Washington, DC, DHHS, 1980.

12. Kramer M: *Psychiatric Services and the Changing Institutional Scene — 1950-1985.* Rockville, MD, National Institute of Mental Health 1977 Series B, No. 12.

13. National Institute of Mental Health: *Patterns in Use of Nursing Homes by the Aged Mentally Ill* Rockville, MD National Institute of Mental Health 1974.

14. Esydlrnki D: The psychogeriatric problem. *Canada's Mental Health* (September 1982) 16-19.

15. Gurland B: Depression and dementia in the elderly of New York City, in *Planning for the Elderly in New York.* New York, Community Council of Greater New York, 1980.

16. Gurland B, Cross PS: Epidemiology of psychopathology in old age. *Psych Clin North Am* 1982: 5(1):11-26.

17. Busse E, Wang HS: The multiple factors contributing to dementia in old age, in *Normal Aging.* Durham, NC, Duke University Press, 1974.

18. Post F: The Factor of Aging in Affective Disorders. *Br J Psychiatry* (Special Publication No. 2) 1968.

19. *The Control of Drugs for the Elderly.* World Health Organization: (EURO Reports and Studies #50) 1981, Copenhagen.

20. Vestal RF: Pharmacology and aging. *J Am Geriatr Soc* 1982; 30(3):191-200.

21. Williamson J, Chopin JM: Adverse reactions to prescribed drugs in the elderly: A multicenter investigation. *Age and Aging* 1980; 9(2):73-80.

22. Drug use and misuse: A growing concern for older Americans (*Joint Hearings Before the Special Committee on Aging, U.S. Senate and Subcommittee on Health and Long Term Care of the Select Committee on Aging, U.S. House of Representatives*). Washington, DC, U.S. Government Printing Office, (HCOA-98-392) June 28, 1983.

23. Levenson AJ: Psychotropic drug use in the elderly: Optimal technique. *Urban Health* (February 1983) 29-31.

24. Bracewell M: Iatrogenic disease in the aged: Physical and mental. Unpublished paper, 1982.

25. *Workshop on Pharmacology & Aging*. Bethesda, MD U.S. Department of Health and Human Services (National Institute of Aging) September, 1977.

26. Buchwald C: *Frequently Prescribed and Abused Drugs*. Brooklyn, NY: Career Teacher Center SUNY, Downstate Medical Center, 1980.

27. Cooper JW: Frequency of potential drug-drug interactions: A seven nursing home study. *J Am Pharm Assoc* 1975; NS515(1):24-31.

28. Reindenberg M: Drugs research and the elderly. *J Hosp Pharm* 1974; 9:210.

29. *National Nursing Home Survey* (Characteristics of Nursing Home Residents, Health Status and Care Received), United States, May-December, 1977; pp 22-89.

30. Ganguli R: The rational use of psychotropic drugs. *Urban Health* (April, 1983) 42-48.

31. *Task Force on Prescription Drugs*. Washington, DC, U.S. Department of Health, Education and Welfare, 1968.

32. Katchthaler T, et al: Incidence of polypharmacy in a long term care facility. *J Am Geriatr Soc* 1977; 25:308.

33. Vancura EJ: Guard against unpredicatable drug responses in the aging. *Geriatrics* (April 1979) 67-73.

34. Crook T, Cohen G: *Physicians' Handbook on Psychotherapeutic Drug Use in the Aged*. New Canaan, CT, Mark Powley Associates, Inc, 1981.

35. Zaske D: Pharmacotherapy: Implications to the elderly. Unpublished paper, 1983.

BIBLIOGRAPHY

Canney M: Determining the Correct Therapeutic Dose. *University of Minnesota Alumni Journal* (October 1983) 6-8.

Cooper JW: Drug therapy in the elderly: Is it all it could be? *American Pharmacy* 1978; NS18(7):25-26.

Glantz MD, et al: *Drugs and the Elderly Adult* (Research Issues 32). DHHS, Rockville, MD, ADAMHA National Institute of Drug Abuse, 1983.

Kidder SW: Saving cost, quality and people: Drug reviews in long-term care. *Am Pharmacy* 1978; NS18(7):18-24.

Pharmaceutical Services in Long-Term Care Facility, 7th ed. Washington, DC, American Health Care Association, 1975.

Drug Metabolism in Elderly Shown Lower. *Today's Nursing Home* (October, 1983) 20-21.

When crushing pills is not appropriate. *Today's Nursing Home* (November 1983) 13-16.

Wedner F: Needed: A comprehensive drug benefit for the elderly. *Am Pharmacy* 1978; NS18(7):28-29.

Chapter 15

ORPHAN DRUG DEVELOPMENT IN GERIATRICS

Marion J. Finkel, MD

Considering the orphan drugs that are well along in the research process or for which new drug applications have been submitted, only one would be used in a disease that is largely, though not exclusively, restricted to the elderly. The sad fact about diseases of the aged is that they are generally not uncommon. Even Alzheimer's disease, formerly thought to be uncommon, has become commonplace due to a clarification of the diagnostic criteria. Looking on the bright side, the frequency of the diseases makes them commercially attractive and not in need of orphan drug development incentives. But sometimes orphan drugs for common disorders do arise when commercial interest is lacking due to unpatentability or imminent patent expiration. Then, too, a given drug may be found useful only for a small subset of an elderly population with a disease, thus consigning it to orphan status.

Therefore, I would like to describe the current status of the federal government's orphan products development program, issues that have arisen as we have been implementing the program, proposed thoughts about their resolution, and whether special studies should be required in elderly patients receiving drugs for uncommon diseases.

There are two definitions of an orphan product — that of the federal government's program and that of the Orphan Drug Act.

In our program we consider not only drugs, but also medical devices, diagnostic products, and medical foods. An orphan product is an unmarketed product for an uncommon condition, or for a common condition where there is no committed commercial sponsor. In addition an orphan indication may exist for a marketed product when there is no committed sponsorship for research and pursuit of labeling for the indication.

The Orphan Drug Act considers only drugs. It defines an orphan drug in economic terms, that is, one intended for a disease or condition so rare in the United States that there is no reasonable expectation that the cost of developing and distributing a drug for such disease or condition will be recovered from U.S. sales of the drug.

Under the act and the government's programs, several incentives are available for conducting research and marketing orphan products. In addition, there are provisions for premarketing availability of orphan drugs to patients.

The act requires the FDA to advise sponsors on the studies needed for marketing approval of orphan drugs. This can be done, at the sponsor's request, prior to and at any time during the clinical development process. Congress intended that the advice rendered would be considered as a commitment by the agency, subject, of course, to revision on the basis of unforeseen circumstances. In September 1983, the FDA issued guidelines for sponsors seeking such advice.

The act also requires the FDA to formally designate drugs as orphan when appropriate. Such designation can be made upon request of a sponsor or on the initiative of the FDA. The FDA has also issued guidelines for sponsors seeking orphan designation. Designation entitles a sponsor to tax credits for the clinical trials undertaken in the United States after designation and prior to marketing approval and to a 7-year exclusive marketing license for an unpatentable drug. As you can imagine, the major incentive of the act is the 7-year exclusive license. This exclusivity is maintained only so long as a sponsor is able to assure the availability of adequate quantities of the drug.

Finally, the act encourages the availability of investigational orphan drugs to physicians and their patients under a treatment IND. Ordinarily, the FDA takes the initiative in suggesting to a firm that it submit a treatment IND. The suggestion is made when the drug is in Phase III, or sometimes Phase II, of development, when the available data demonstrate that the drug is probably safe and effective, and when the drug serves as an important alternative to other available therapy.

A major incentive for orphan drug development is provided by the grant and contract mechanism. The federal government supports orphan product research and has done so for many years, although such support was not heretofore defined in orphan terms. Recently, the National Institutes of Health invited the submission of grant applications for orphan product research and the National Institute of Neurological and Communicative Disorders and Stroke announced that it had set aside some funds for contracts. The FDA recently awarded 12 grants and issued another call for applications in January of 1984. By government regulation, grants and contracts are available to applicants from both nonprofit and for-profit institutions.

The federal government offers still another incentive — that is, it can grant to a drug company exclusive rights to preclinical and clinical data generated under government support in return for agreement by the company to complete development of, and to market, an orphan product.

The FDA's orphan products development program is not only reactive but proactive, that is, it provides advice and makes orphan drug designations upon request, but it also seeks out new products, both in this country and abroad, considers the award of contracts to complete research needed for marketing approval, and obtains commitments from companies to market the products.

Despite the incentives described there are still potential obstacles in the path of orphan product development. One of these is the issue of liability and this may be of particular concern with a geriatric population prone to major organ dysfunction and the ingestion of many drugs in addition to the orphan drug. The Orphan Products Board of the Department of Health and Human Services recently reviewed the question of whether liability serves as a disincentive to orphan product development. It concluded that, in general, it does not although it may be a factor in isolated instances. Nevertheless, the board is watching the situation closely and will consider what solutions are available should the need arise.

Another potential obstacle is the relative lack of support for the animal toxicology studies required for clinical research and marketing approval. NIH grants sometimes cover both preclinical and clinical studies; the FDA's laboratories have indicated a willingness to perform animal studies on occasion; and the Pharmaceutical Manufacturers Association's Commission on Drugs for Rare Diseases has sought the support of specific studies by member firms or other interested parties, but these sources will not eliminate the problem. Grant and contract appropriations under the Orphan Drug Act must be applied only to clinical trials. The Orphan Products Board and academicians whose research is stalled by the lack of animal toxicology studies are considering methods for increasing the amount of available support.

Another obstacle is the perception by companies that data requirements for marketing approval of orphan drugs are similar to those for drugs intended for large patient populations. The standards for approval are the same (ie, orphan drugs must be shown to be safe and effective by means of adequate and well-controlled studies), but the volume, extent, and nature of the studies are tailored to the specific orphan disease. To illustrate, I would like to describe the data that supported a recently approved orphan drug.

Acetohydroxamic acid is used as adjunctive therapy in patients who have chronic or repetitive urinary tract infections caused by urea-splitting organisms. These infections result in elevated ammonia and pH levels in the urine and, often, the formation of struvite stones. The drug inhibits the bacterial enzyme urease, which is responsible for the formation of excess ammonia levels in the urine, and lessens the likelihood of stone formation. Paraplegics and patients with congenital or acquired anatomical defects of the urinary tract constitute major groups prone to urinary tract infections from urea-splitting organisms.

For the preclinical data, the sponsor of the new drug application submitted published reports of acute toxicity studies, a small subacute study in dogs performed in his laboratory, and a carcinogenicity study in rats performed by an investigator in partial fulfillment of his PhD requirements. The subacute and carcinogenicity studies were not of the type performed today and were not designed, as they are today, to provide complete information on toxicity as well. Nevertheless, they provided some basic information on potential adverse effects, particularly the subacute study in dogs.

The clinical data consisted of a double-blind, placebo-controlled trial, an open study of nonrandomized but concomitantly followed treated and untreated groups, and a published study that used historical controls and, in some patients, a positive control.

A total of about 100 patients received the investigational drug. The investigators were able to show a difference in the occurrence or rate of progression of stone growth between drug-treated and untreated or placebo-treated patients.

In this case there were three studies. It is quite likely that had the investigations begun with the double-blind, randomized, placebo-controlled trial, two studies alone would have sufficed, or perhaps even one, had the well controlled study been expanded to a multiclinic trial. This is because the principal investigator had laid the groundwork for his clinical trials by the performance of sophisticated studies demonstrating the pharmacologic effect of the drug in patients and experimental animals. In addition, because there had been considerable interest in this compound and others of its class for years, there was a significant amount of published data on its pharmacologic effects.

The question can be asked whether special studies would have been required in the elderly. Because orphan diseases are generally rare diseases, the chances are small of including an elderly population in the clinical trials of sufficient size to provide meaningful data in this age group. If an orphan disease affects the elderly as well as other age groups, however, one would want to consider the desirability of at least determining, when appropriate, the effect of renal dysfunction on the rate of clearance of the drug. As a minimum the labeling should warn, when appropriate, that initial doses should be lower in the elderly until individual patient response can be determined.

If an orphan drug is intended exclusively or almost exclusively for the elderly, there may be a sufficient number of patients available in the clinical trials to perform some special pharmacokinetic studies. The specific studies to be done will, of course, depend upon the nature of the drug.

In summary, the requirements of marketing approval of an orphan drug are basically similar to those for a commercial drug; adequate evidence of safety and effectiveness based on well controlled studies. Animal toxicologic requirements and the number and size of the clinical trials are tailored to the individual circumstances. When an orphan drug is to be used largely in a geriatric population, special studies of its safety relative to use in the elderly should be considered.

Chapter 16

GERIATRIC DRUG RESEARCH IN THE VETERANS ADMINISTRATION

Robert E. Vestal, MD
Robert E. Allen, PhD

The purpose of this paper is threefold: (1) to emphasize the impact on the Veterans Administration (VA) health care delivery system of the demographic shift in the United States toward an increasingly aged population, (2) to provide an overview of the VA Research and Development Program, and (3) to indicate the level of VA research activity devoted to aging and geriatric pharmacology.

IMPACT OF AGING VETERAN POPULATION

Recent statistics from the U.S. Census Bureau indicate that in 1982 26.8 million Americans, 11.7% of the population, were 65 years of age or older. By 2030 that number will increase to 64.3 million and will account for more than 21% of the population. The VA has reason for special concern as World War II veterans enter the geriatric age group (Figure 16.1). The veteran population aged 65 years and older expressed as a percentage of the general population in this age group will increase from 10.6% in 1980 to 37% in the year 2000 as compared to an increase from 11.3% to only 12.2% in the general population (Figure 16.2). An even more impressive way to express these data is to show the number of veterans over 65 years as a percent of all American males over 65 years of age (Figure 16.3). In 1976 about 24% of men over age 65 were veterans. This will increase to 60% by the year 2000.

VA RESEARCH AND DEVELOPMENT PROGRAM

Although there has been a gradual increase in the numbers of investigators in the VA Research and Development Program, from 4,253 in 1979 to 5,868 in 1983 (an increase of 38%), the research and development budget

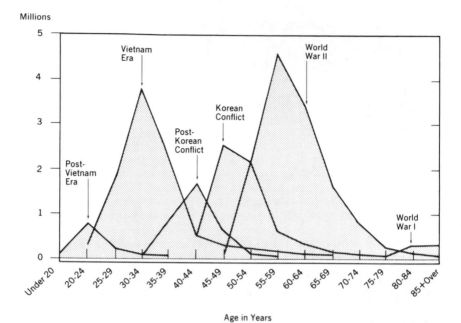

Figure 16.1. Graph of Veterans Administration data showing number of veterans in various age groups since World War I.

as a percentage of the total medical care budget has declined 8% during the same period of time. This is a disappointing message, particularly during an era when two VA investigators received the Nobel Prize in Medicine. Nevertheless, this increase in the number of investigators emphasizes the attractiveness to academic physicians of research opportunities in the VA.

Funding allocated to the VA Research and Development Program, $154 million in 1983 (Table 16.1), is small by comparison to the nearly $4 billion budget of the National Institutes of Health. It is important to emphasize, however, that salaries of clinician-investigators are not included in these figures, that no overhead is paid, and that many clinical studies can be performed with very modest budgets.

The majority of the budget is used by programs in Medical Research Service, but there was a much needed increase in the allocation for rehabilitative research in 1983. It is also noteworthy that during the period from 1979 to 1983 there was approximately a 75% increase in extra-VA funding awarded to VA investigators. Support awarded to the VA investigators by the National Institute on Aging (NIA) increased by 145% during the same period. This indicates that more VA investigators are seeking extramural support for aging research and that they are successful in competing for those funds.

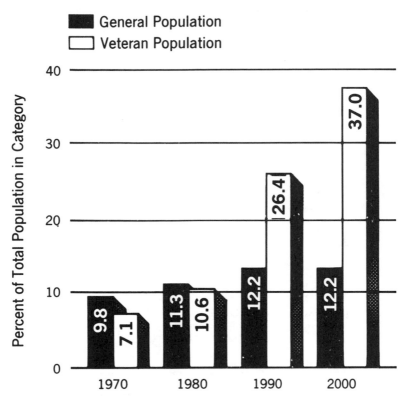

Figure 16.2. Percentage of population 65 or older, general population and veterans 1970 through 2000. Source: Office of Reports and Statistics, VA Central Office, April 1983.

Mechanisms of intramural VA support for research on aging are listed in Table 16.2. The central focus of VA research is the Merit Review Program. This is a program based on investigator-initiated proposals. These proposals are reviewed by Merit Review Boards, of which there are 15 devoted to various fields of investigation in medicine and biology. Approximately half of the board members are VA investigators and half are non-VA investigators. The Merit Review Boards are equivalent to the NIH Study Sections and proposals are reviewed with equivalent rigor. Members of the boards often serve or have served on NIH Study Sections.

A major category of aging research in the VA is research conducted under the auspices of the Geriatric Research, Education and Clinical Centers (the GRECCs). There are now 10 such centers in the country, including the newly established programs at the Durham, North Carolina VA Medical Center and Gainesville, Florida VA Medical Center. Each GRECC has one or two

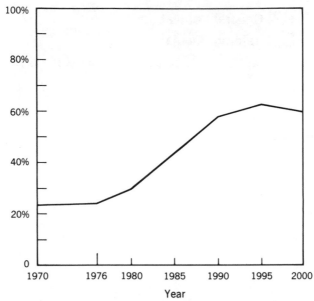

Figure 16.3. Veterans over 65 years as percentage of all U.S. males over 65 years of age, 1970 through 2000.

Table 16.1. Research in the Veterans Administration

	FY 1979	FY 1980	FY 1981	FY 1982	FY 1983
Investigators	4253	4185	5108	5407	5868
VAMC with centrally allocated R&D funding	118	123	126	122	123
R&D/medical care budget (%)	2.20	2.16	2.12	1.92	2.03
R&D budget ($ millions)	122	125	140	141	154
Medical research	113	115	128	131	141
Rehabilitative research	6	7	9	7	10
Health services	3	3	3	3	3
Extra-VA funding ($ millions)	34.4	42.0	50.7	47.8	61.4
NIA	0.48	0.65	0.99	1.05	1.18

major foci of research activity. For example, the Gainesville GRECC will emphasize geropharmacology. The GRECC investigators must also compete for research support through the Merit Review Program, but as described below they currently enjoy a favored status. The Cooperative Studies Program

Table 16.2. Mechanisms of Support in the VA for Research on Aging

Merit Review Program
Geriatric Research, Education and Clinical Centers (GRECC)
  High Priority (Aging — 106G)
Cooperative Studies Program
Career Development Program
Geriatric Physician Fellowship Research Program
Innovative Aging Program

is a very well known program in the VA. One of the currently supported projects focuses on the treatment of mild hypertension in the elderly. The Career Development Program supports investigators at several levels in their academic careers and is similar to the NIH Research Career Development Program. Recently, the Geriatric Physician Fellowship Research Program has been added and is supported through the Office of Academic Affairs, which is the educational arm of the VA. This program provides a third year to physicians in the Geriatric Clinical Fellowship Program who want to obtain research experience.

There are two unique features in the way research is funded through the VA. As indicated by Figure 16.4, Merit Review Research Programs with priority scores of 34 or better receive funding. Approved programs with priority scores of 35 or worse are not funded. Programs with priority scores between 10 and 15 receive the full budget approved by the Merit Review Board. Programs with priority scores between 15 and 34 receive a variable percentage of the approved budget (see Figure 16.4). Unlike the situation with NIH grants, VA programs approved with priority scores of 34 or better on the basis of scientific merit receive at least some support. In addition, aging has been identified as a high priority area. Approved research programs dealing with aging, which are submitted by GRECC or GRECC-affiliated investigators, receive full funding provided that the priority score is 34 or better.

The majority of research programs in the VA are in the category of Merit Review (Table 16.3). Thus, the bulk of support goes to investigator-initiated proposals. There has been an increase in high priority research over the past 5 years. As previously stated, this category enjoys favored status in terms of funding and includes aging research. Other areas of particular relevance to veterans fall within the high priority category also. The number of Cooperative Studies Programs has remained relatively constant while there was an unfortunate decline in the Career Development Program until 1983. The Research Advisory Group Program has also suffered a decline. These trends are particularly distressing because these are the programs that support newly recruited VA investigators.

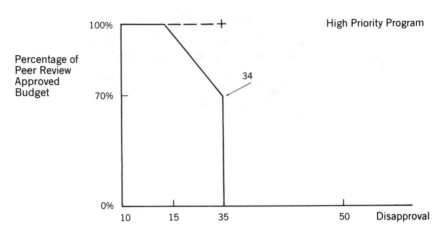

Figure 16.4. Priority funding of GRECC research.

Table 16.3. Number of Funded VA Research Programs

Program	FY 1979	FY 1980	FY 1981	FY 1982	FY 1983
Merit Review	1,514	1,515	1,566	1,494	1,819
High Priority	37	81	87	93	124
Aging (106G)	37	35	42	40	33
Cooperative Studies	27	26	22	24	25
Career Development	200	186	185	122	210
Research Advisory Group	254	229	210	193	199

RESEARCH ON AGING AND GERIATRIC PHARMACOLOGY IN THE VA

Turning specifically to the issue of aging research, it is important to first emphasize that the method used to track research activity depends on the investigator's own identification of his/her primary and/or secondary *program* areas. It is also important to recognize that the investigator's program may include several *projects,* which may or may not be related. For example, an investigator's program may have one project devoted to aging, but four other projects not related to aging. Therefore, he/she may not identify aging as the primary program area and may not even identify it as a secondary program area.

Table 16.4 lists by year the numbers of principal investigators who identified aging as either a primary or a secondary program area. Funding is also indicated. There has been a substantial increase in the number of principal investigator's reporting in these areas, from 186 in 1979 to 333 in 1983. Thus, approximately 18% of VA Merit Review programs are currently conducting research related to aging.

Table 16.4. Research on Aging*

Fiscal	Primary Program Area		Secondary Program Area		Total	
	Number of PIs	Funding ($ millions)	Number of PIs	Funding ($ millions)	Number of PIs	Funding* ($ millions)
1977		1.4 (0.4)**				
1978		1.7 (0.8)				
1979	78	1.8 (1.1)	108	4.4	186	6.2
1980	104	2.4 (1.2)	122	5.1	226	7.5
1981	113	2.9 (1.5)	131	5.9	244	8.8
1982	139	3.1 (1.7)	153	6.2	292	9.3
1983	169	3.2 (1.8)	164	6.6	333	9.8

*Calculations do not include salaries for clinical investigators.
**Within GRECC Program.

It is difficult to determine in a precise way the extent to which pharmacology and aging are combined in the programs of VA investigators. Although in 1983 a significant number of investigators listed aging or clinical pharmacology as primary or secondary program areas, only nine investigators listed *both* aging and clinical pharmacology (Table 16.5). Two of these investigators were at the Boise VA Medical Center; that number has increased to five in the past year. The point is, of course, that not many investigators in the country consider themselves to be gerontological pharmacologists. Indeed, the Boise VA Medical Center has the only geriatric clinical pharmacology unit in the VA system, and it is fortunate to receive research support from both intramural and extramural sources. The above figures underestimate, however, the level of activity. As of March 1983, 440 investigators with centrally funded research programs listed 469 project titles related to aging. Of these 440 investigators, based on project title, 40 (9.1%) had a project related to both aging and pharmacology. This means that in 1983 about 2.2% of VA projects funded in Merit Review are doing some work in relation to aging and pharmacology. These projects are focused on pharmacokinetics, pharmacodynamics, the autonomic nervous system, drug treatment of Alzheimer's disease, hypertension in the elderly, age-related behavioral and biochemical effects of alcohol, and anesthesia and aging, to give a few examples.

Finally, a brief comment should be made about the Innovative Aging Program. This is a new VA program initiated in October 1983, with solicitation in December 1982, of proposals for research studies dealing with biological processes underlying aging. There were 354 letters of intent to apply and, ultimately, there were 200 proposals, of which 135 were approved for scientific review. Of those, 57% were approved by the scientific peer review panels.

Table 16.5. Program Area Designations in Aging
or Clinical Pharmacology

Program Area	Number of Investigators (FY 1983)	Total VA Funding ($ millions)
Primary program area*		
Aging	169	3.2
Clinical pharmacology	90	1.7
Secondary program area**		
Aging	164	6.6
Clinical pharmacology	127	3.5
Totals		
Aging**	333	9.8
Clinical pharmacology	217	5.2

*Only nine investigators listed both aging and clinical pharmacology as primary and secondary program areas.

**Including centrally funded research for FY 1983 as of March, 1983, 440 investigators listed 469 project titles related to aging. Of these 440 investigators, based on the title, 40 (9.1%) had a project related to both aging and pharmacology.

Unfortunately, only 18 projects or 13% could be funded. These 2-year projects have a maximum funding level of $50,000 per year. Of these 18 funded projects, 6 or 33% addressed topics related to aging and pharmacology. The topic areas were as follows: (1) blood-brain barrier permeability, (2) culture of central cholinergic and aminergic neurons, (3) microsomal hepatic drug metabolism, (4) molecular forms of acetylcholinesterase in skeletal muscle, (5) muscarinic receptor binding in vitro, and (6) angiotensin receptors.

SUMMARY

It is evident that the VA faces a challenge as it seeks to address the needs of an increasingly aged veteran population. A number of clinical, educational, and research programs have been established to meet this challenge. Efforts to provide increased funding levels for aging research have included the establishment of aging as a high priority research area and the Innovative Aging Program. Relatively few VA investigators identify themselves as having programs in gerontological pharmacology, but it is likely that they will gradually increase in numbers.

Chapter 17

GERIATRIC DRUG RESEARCH AT NIH AND ADAMHA

George M. Steinberg

This chapter contains a discussion of geriatric drug research at NIH and ADAMHA including all elements of pharmacology, not simply drug usage and drug effects. There will be emphasis on three aspects: (1) program objectives, (2) the magnitude and distribution of resources, and (3) the function of administrators in program development.

The elderly in the United States are already a large segment of the population and their numbers are increasing rapidly. Those over 65 years of age now comprise 11% to 12% of the population. In 50 years, that figure may increase to 17% to 20%. NIA's objectives are to provide information that will aid in the improved use of existing drugs in elderly patients and that will contribute to the development of improved drugs in the future. It is also important to develop improved strategies for treating diseases that principally affect the elderly.

In an absolute sense, elderly people do not respond to drugs differently than younger adults. Differences, where they exist, are quantitative, not qualitative. They are differences in degree only. I prefer to refer to them as alterations in responses rather than differences. Alterations have been observed. Various physiological functions and body composition change with aging so that alterations in drug response are not unexpected. Alterations

---

Abbreviations: NIH: National Institutes of Health; NIA: National Institute on Aging; NIADDK: National Institute on Arthritis, Diabetes, and Digestive and Kidney Diseases; NCI: National Cancer Institute; NEI: National Eye Institute; NICHD: National Institute of Child Health and Human Development; NHLBI: National Heart, Lung, and Blood Institute; NINCDS: National Institute of Neurological and Communicative Disorders and Stroke; DRR: Division of Research Resources. ADAMHA: Alcohol, Drug Abuse and Mental Health Administration. NIAAA: National Institute on Alcohol Abuse and Alcoholism; NIDA: National Institute on Drug Abuse; NIMH: National Institute of Mental Health. *NIH Guide: NIH Guide to Grants and Contracts.*

in response may occur either for desired drug effects, for undesired side effects, or for both. It has been suggested that the elderly are more subject to side effects. Whether this generalization is true remains uncertain because most reports have been criticized for inadequate experimental design. Further, where increased sensitivity has been reported, the authors have often not corrected for altered pharmacokinetics through appropriately corrected dosage. Thus, we do not have a solid body of information on alterations in pharmacodynamics that occur with aging. Nonetheless, despite the paucity of scientific proof, there are reasons to believe that the elderly are at higher risk to adverse drug effects. They seem to exhibit a greater sensitivity to many drugs, particularly those that act on the central nervous system. Because of a greater incidence of multiple pathology and multiple drug use in elderly patients there is also greater chance for drug-drug and drug-disease interactions.

We believe that the drug developers, primarily the pharmaceutical manufacturers, are in the best position to define alterations in pharmacokinetics and in responsiveness of elderly patients to individual drugs. Such information can be obtained most readily during preapproval clinical studies by adding elderly subjects to drug trials. It should be noted, however, that elderly patients show a greater range of drug responsiveness than younger patients, so large numbers of elderly subjects may have to be included. We believe that the Federal Government can contribute most effectively by concentrating on identifying aging-related alterations in pharmacodynamics and determining the mechanistic alterations responsible. Such information should contribute to the improved use of existing drugs and should be important for the development of new drugs that give superior therapy or act prophylactically to prevent the diseases found in old age. Another important area for federal research is the development of pharmaceutical agents for diseases that presently have no effective drug therapy, as, for example, Alzheimer's disease and benign prostatic hypertrophy.

Federally supported research projects in pharmacology that deal with aging processes or with aging-related diseases and disabilities cover a wide range of scientific topics. Examples of the more active areas are given in Table 17.1.

Table 17.1. NIH and ADAMHA Research Projects
in Gerontological Pharmacology

Area	No. of Projects
Alzheimer's disease and other dementias	22
Cognition, memory, depression	11
Catecholamines	9
Anesthesia	6
Alcoholism	5

Within the NIH and ADAMHA, support is widely distributed. Indicated in Table 17.2 is the level of support provided in FY 1983 for extramural research by Institutes that are part of NIH and ADAMHA. For comparison, the number of corresponding intramural research projects is given in Table 17.3. Extramural research is that carried out at laboratories not administratively managed by the funding agency. Research support provided to these laboratories is generally in the form of grants-in-aid. These provide major but not complete support for individual research projects. Most laboratories that receive extramural support are university-based or in other non-profit organizations. However, they also include other government laboratories, such as those of the Veterans Administration, and may include for-profit organizations. Intramural laboratories are directly supported and administratively managed by individual Institutes. It is noteworthy that approximately 95% of the projects supported in FY 1983 were carried out in extramural laboratories.

Table 17.2. Extramural Projects (FY 1983) in Gerontological Pharmacology

Agency	No. of Projects	$ (millions)
National Institutes of Health		
NIA	91	7.5
NIADDK	4	.4
NCI	1	.01
NEI	3	.2
NICHD	1	.04
NHLBI	18	3.5
NINCDS	8	.65
DRR	34	.75
Alcohol, Drug Abuse and Mental Health Administration		
NIAAA	5	.65
NIDA	1	.2
NIMH	25	2.9
Total	191	16.8

Table 17.3. Intramural Projects (FY 1983) in Gerontological Pharmacology

Agency		No. of Projects
NIH		
	NIA	8
	NEI	2
ADAMHA		
	NIMH	1

In Table 17.2, one can see that the major support is provided by NIA, but that NHLBI and NIMH are also large supporters. One may also note that support is distributed among virtually all of the Institutes. Such a spread is normal and is to be expected. It results from the normal overlap in Institute responsibilities and program areas. For example, should a grant that contrasts cardiac function in young adults and in elderly persons be assigned to NHLBI or NIA?

The scientific areas under study in gerontological pharmacology are diverse. Data taken from our computer files do not distinguish projects that are entirely devoted to gerontological pharmacology from those in which it is a significant but minor component. Hence, the total sum of $16.8 million represents a somewhat inflated estimate of the funds applied to aging. While there are a large number of projects being supported, many fall outside areas that are identified for concentration of effort.

It may be of value at this point to outline briefly the NIH (and ADAM-HA) method for administering grant applications. Most grant applications are investigator-initiated research proposals. These are reviewed for scientific merit by peer review panels, which are completely independent of the Institute administrators. There is much merit in such a process, since it provides opportunities for new and original ideas and does not limit evaluative judgments to single individuals. However, it is one of the functions of Institute scientific administrators to help concentrate community efforts in addressing pressing biomedical issues. We do this in several ways, calling upon leading members of the scientific community wherever possible. For example, we organize meetings to openly discuss important research topics before interested audiences. We hold limited participation workshops with panels of experts for the development of statements of research needs in areas where little work is being done. In either case, we arrange to have the reports and recommendations published in widely read scientific journals. This information helps grant applicants in their development of new proposals and review groups in their evaluative processes since degree of scientific need is one of the criteria used in making judgments.

Table 17.4 outlines the priority research needs identified in a workshop held by the NIA pharmacology program several years ago. The group's recommendations were wide-ranging. Some of their recommendations fall within the scope of the pharmacology program and some into those of other NIA programs. (More detailed information on the conclusions of the workshop is provided in Reference 1.)

NIA program initiatives are under way in several of the suggested areas including Alzheimer's disease, urinary incontinence, and hypertension. For Alzheimer's disease and urinary incontinence there have been workshops and *NIH Guide* announcements. Shortly, in collaboration with NHLBI, we will undertake a large-scale, multicentered clinical trial on the treatment of isolated systolic hypertension in the aged. Hypertension in the elderly is often characterized by an elevated systolic pressure and a normal diastolic pressure. In this trial, we will determine if reduction of elevated systolic pressure

Table 17.4. Research Needs in Gerontological Pharmacology

---

1. Drug actions on the cardiovascular system and the peripheral and central nervous systems
2. Effects of drugs and modulators on the immune system and on bone metabolism
3. Prevention and treatment of common diseases and disorders of the elderly including Alzheimer's disease and other dementias, osteoporosis, osteoarthritis, urinary incontinence, altered response to treatment of infection, hypertension/hypotension, cancer, and decubitus ulcers
4. Clinical and basic pharmacological research to identify mechanisms involved in altered drug responses in the elderly

---

will reduce the incidence of mortality and morbidity, principally nonfatal strokes, in an elderly population.

The NIA pharmacology program is in the process of developing a number of program initiatives. I will refer to two of them in greater detail to provide a sense of how administrators shape a program.

The first program initiative covers blood pressure regulation and aging processes. Hypertension is one of the more important diseases of the elderly. It is estimated that more than 40% of those aged over 65 have this disorder. Because of the damage it produces in such organs as the heart, brain, and kidney, hypertension is a major contributor to disease of the elderly. In the elderly, hypertension is expressed somewhat differently than in younger adults. Often there is a disproportionately high systolic pressure, and wide swings in pressure are not uncommon. Inadequate blood pressure response in the elderly sometimes leads to hypotensive episodes. Altered responses are believed to be related to reduced aortic distensibility, increased peripheral vascular resistance, and blunted baroreceptor sensitivity. However, the study of these and other pathophysiological factors has been limited and the opportunity exists for in-depth investigation.

Currently only one project has been identified that addresses this issue. Our program, which we are carrying out in collaboration with NHLBI, was initiated last year. At a workshop planning session held with a small group of leading researchers, we developed a plan for a meeting to be held later this year. In developing the workshop plan, we determined questions to be addressed, decided on scientific disciplines and people required, and developed a format that will provide a focus for the meeting and produce a balanced report. There will be about 30 participants at the workshop. A full report including background papers and recommendations will be published in a major biomedical journal. In addition, we will further alert the biomedical research community by publishing a program announcement in the *NIH Guide*. We anticipate that these activities will result in a considerable increase in research activity.

The second program initiative is on catecholamines and aging processes. The sympathetic nervous system is involved in the homeostatic regulation of a wide variety of central and peripheral functions. Agents that mimic or alter its activity are used to treat disorders such as hypertension, shock, cardiac failure, arrhythmias, asthma, allergy, anaphylaxis, depression, anxiety, and psychosis. In addition, age-associated changes in catecholaminergic regulation have been implicated in several disorders of the elderly, including Alzheimer's disease, sleep disorders, and syncope.

Currently, the annual support level for such research at NIH and ADAMHA is $1.5 million. This covers a fair range of subjects. Most of the studies are in animals, and much more research, particularly in humans, is needed. For example, there has been a modest amount of research on the response to beta-agonists and -antagonists. It seems that there is a decrease in responsiveness with aging. Whether this is due to reduced receptor sensitivity, reduced receptor number, or to other factors is a matter of controversy. Whether the reduction in responsiveness is organ-specific also remains to be determined. Preliminary studies suggest that this may be so. A major question is why blood norepinephrine levels are elevated in the elderly. The effect of aging on the response to alpha-agonists and -antagonists has received almost no attention. Last year, we held a symposium on "Aging and Drugs which Affect Noradrenergic Systems in Man." A first draft of the summary paper has been prepared and should be published by mid-1984. Also, we plan to hold a planning session for a comprehensive workshop on "Catecholamines and Aging Processes" to be held in 1985.

This will be followed by a comprehensive report to be published in a major biomedical journal and also an *NIH Guide* program announcement. Similar plans on the subjects of microcirculation and anesthesia are at an earlier stage of development.

In summary, drug research for the elderly at NIH and ADAMHA is carried out principally by the NIA. It also receives considerable support from NHLBI and NIMH and to a lesser extent from most of the other Institutes. Most of the funds support extramural projects.

The major thrust of drug research for the elderly is to increase understanding of the nature and causes of alterations in drug responses, particularly on the cardiovascular and nervous systems, and to develop new and improved means for treating diseases that principally affect the elderly.

REFERENCE

1. Steinberg GM, Schneider, EL: NIA Second Workshop on Pharmacology and Aging, June 1981. *The Pharmacologist* 1982; 24:65–67.

PART 7

RISK FACTORS IN GERIATRIC DRUG USE

Chapter 18

DRUG INTERACTIONS IN GERIATRIC DRUG USE

Daniel A. Hussar

The term *drug interaction* is applied most frequently to those situations in which the effects of one drug are altered by the prior or concurrent use of another (drug-drug interactions). It should also be recognized that the effects of drugs or nutrients may be affected by the action of the other (drug-nutrient interactions), that drugs may interfere with laboratory test results (drug-laboratory test interactions), and that some drugs may be more likely to cause unwanted effects in patients with certain disease states (drug-disease interactions). Although these types of interactions are also important, this discussion will focus on the factors concerning the development of drug-drug interactions in elderly patients.

FACTORS CONTRIBUTING TO THE OCCURRENCE OF DRUG INTERACTIONS

Multiple Pharmacologic Effects

Most drugs used in current therapy do not just possess one specific type of activity, but have the capacity to influence many physiologic systems. Therefore, two concomitantly administered drugs will often affect some of the same systems. When considering the potential for interactions between drugs there is often a tendency to be concerned only with the primary effects of the drugs involved and to overlook the secondary activities they possess. Combined therapy with a phenothiazine antipsychotic (eg, chlorpromazine [Thorazine]), a tricyclic antidepressant (eg, amitriptyline [Elavil]), and an antiparkinson agent (eg, trihexyphenidyl [Artane]) is frequently employed. Each of these agents has a considerably different primary effect; however, all three possess anticholinergic activity, characterized by symptoms such as dryness of the mouth and blurring of vision. Even though the anticholinergic effect of any one of the drugs may be slight, the additive effects of the three agents may be significant.

Many health professionals might consider an effect such as dryness of mouth as a minor problem; however, it can be especially troublesome in certain elderly patients. For example, persistent dryness of the mouth could make the use of dentures more difficult and also cause other dental complications; in addition, there may be increased difficulty in chewing and swallowing, an important factor with respect to the problem of malnutrition in many elderly individuals. A recent case report of a patient treated with imipramine (Tofranil) described another potential problem. The patient experienced persistent dryness of the mouth and, when nitroglycerin tablets were administered sublingually for the management of exertional angina, the relief of the symptoms was delayed because of the slower dissolution of the sublingual tablets.

It has also been observed that an excessive anticholinergic effect can cause an atropine-like delirium, and geriatric patients are at the greatest risk of such a response. This effect could be mistaken as a worsening of the conditions being treated and might be managed by increasing the dosage of the therapeutic agents. This example points out the difficulty that can often exist in distinguishing between the symptoms of the clinical disorder(s) and the effects of the drug(s) being employed as therapy.

Additional observations concerning the concurrent use of antipsychotic agents and antiparkinson agents merit further study. Several reports have described the development of severe hyperpyrexia in patients taking such combinations who were exposed to high environmental temperature and humidity. These investigators call attention to the ability of these combinations to interfere with the thermoregulatory system of the body and recommend that patients who are receiving high doses of these agents should minimize exposure to hot and humid conditions.

Multiple Physicians

It is necessary for some individuals to go to more than one physician, and it is not uncommon for a patient to be seeing one or more specialists in addition to a family physician. It is frequently difficult for one physician to learn completely what medications have been prescribed for a patient by another physician, and many difficulties could arise from such situations. For example, one physician may prescribe an antihistamine for a patient for whom another physician has prescribed an antianxiety agent with the possible consequence of an excessive depressant effect.

Even though the patient is seeing different physicians, he or she will usually have the prescriptions filled at the same pharmacy. Therefore, the pharmacist, by maintaining patient medication records, can play an important role in the detection and prevention of drug-related problems.

Concurrent Use of Prescription and Nonprescription Drugs

Many reports of drug interactions have involved the concurrent use of a prescription drug with a nonprescription drug (eg, aspirin, antacids, antihistamines, decongestants). When physicians question patients about medications that they are taking, patients will often neglect to mention the nonprescription medications they have purchased. Many patients have been taking preparations such as antacids, analgesics, and iron preparations for such long periods or in such a routine manner that they do not consider them to be drugs. This information can be easily missed in casually questioning a patient, and some physicians and pharmacists prefer to utilize a list of symptoms that might ordinarily be treated with nonprescription drugs in trying to obtain this information from the patient.

Although many individuals will have their prescriptions filled in their local pharmacy, they often purchase nonprescription drugs elsewhere, thus making identification of potential problems extremely difficult for the pharmacist as well as the physician. For this reason, patients should be encouraged to obtain both their prescription and nonprescription medications at the same pharmacy. However, such advice is justified only when the pharmacist personally supervises the sale of nonprescription medications with which problems may develop.

Patient Noncompliance

For a variety of reasons many patients do not take medication according to directions. A number of patients have not received adequate instructions from the physician and pharmacist as to how and when to take their medication. In some other situations, particularly involving those patients who are taking several medications, confusion about the instructions may develop even though the patient may have understood them initially.

It is easy to understand how the geriatric patient who may be taking five or six medications several times a day at different times can become confused or forget to take his or her medication, although these occurrences are by no means unique to the geriatric population.

Although the situations involving noncompliance would usually result in a patient not taking enough medication, some circumstances could lead to the excessive use of certain medications, thereby increasing the possibility of drug interaction. For example, some patients who realize they have forgotten a dose of medication double the next dose to make up for it. Other patients apparently subscribe to a philosophy that if the one-tablet dose that has been prescribed provides some relief of symptoms, two or three tablets will be even more effective.

CONSEQUENCES OF DRUG INTERACTIONS

Drug interactions are often viewed as a type of adverse drug reaction and, indeed, one of the most important consequences of a drug interaction is an excessive response to one or both of the agents being utilized. A significantly enhanced effect of agents like warfarin and digoxin can result in serious complications, and the hazards of combining agents having central nervous system depressant properties are also well known. Not as well recognized, but also very important, are those interactions in which drug activity is decreased, resulting in a loss of efficacy. These interactions are especially difficult to detect, since they may be mistaken for therapeutic failure or progression of the disease.

It should also be recognized that sometimes a second drug is prescribed deliberately to modify the effects of another. Such an approach might be utilized in an effort to enhance the effectiveness or to reduce the adverse effects of the primary agent. In these situations, the efficacy and/or safety of a drug is increased, indicating that drug interactions are not always harmful, as frequently thought, but can also be beneficial.

Although some drug interactions develop unexpectedly and are impossible to predict, others are related to known pharmacodynamic and pharmacokinetic properties of the drugs and can be reasonably anticipated. However, in considering the complex nature of the agents utilized in many multiple-drug regimens, the ability to predict the magnitude of a specific action of any given drug diminishes. These circumstances point to a need not only for maintenance of complete and current medication records for patients, but also for closer monitoring and supervision of drug therapy so that problems can be prevented or detected at an early stage in their development.

INCREASED RISK OF INTERACTIONS IN THE ELDERLY

The methodologies employed in the few comprehensive studies that have been conducted have varied considerably and, for this and other reasons, the presently available data must be viewed as inconclusive with respect to the incidence of interactions. However, a number of factors clearly point to an increased risk in the elderly. Most elderly patients have at least one chronic illness (eg, hypertension, diabetes) and this is reflected in the prescribing of a larger number of medications for this patient group. The types of diseases more frequently experienced by geriatric patients (eg, renal disorders) may contribute to an altered drug response, and there appears to be an increased sensitivity to the action of certain drugs with advancing age. In addition, there may be age-related changes in the absorption, distribution, metabolism, and excretion of certain drugs that increase the possibility of adverse drug reactions and drug interactions. Accordingly, drug therapy in geriatric patients must be monitored especially closely.

MECHANISMS OF DRUG INTERACTION

The list of reported drug interactions is too long to try to commit them all to memory. However, an understanding of the mechanisms by which these interactions develop will be valuable in anticipating such situations and dealing with problems that do develop. Although the circumstances surrounding the development of some drug interactions are complex and poorly understood, the mechanisms by which many interactions develop are well documented and relate to the basic processes by which a drug acts and is acted upon in the body.

These mechanisms are often generally categorized as being of pharmacokinetic and pharmacodynamic types. Pharmacokinetic interactions are those in which the absorption, distribution, metabolism, or excretion (ADME) of a drug is altered. Included among the pharmacodynamic interactions are those in which drugs having similar (or opposing) pharmacological effects are administered concurrently and situations in which the sensitivity or responsiveness of the tissues to one drug is altered by another. Although the pharmacokinetic interactions often present challenging clinical problems, which have been widely publicized, the pharmacodynamic interactions are more frequently encountered. It should also be recognized that several mechanisms may be involved in the development of certain interactions.

The influence of the aging process on certain of the mechanisms through which drug interactions develop has been described in a number of studies. Elevated gastric pH, a reduction in intestinal blood flow, and decreased gastrointestinal motility are often associated with aging, although the alterations of absorption that result appear to be less important than other age-related factors that affect drug action.

The distribution of certain drugs may be altered as total body water and extracellular fluid decrease with age, whereas the proportion of body fat increases. Therefore, there may be higher blood levels in the elderly of those agents that are distributed primarily in body water, whereas the age-associated changes may result in an increased volume of distribution, and lower blood levels, of other agents.

There appears to be an age-related decline in the efficiency of the oxidative metabolic pathways, suggesting that there will also be a decline in the extent to which these metabolic processes are affected by therapeutic agents. Conjugation pathways, however, appear to function with comparable efficiency irrespective of age. There is also an age-related reduction of hepatic blood flow and this may contribute to a reduced rate of metabolism of certain agents and an increased incidence of adverse effects in the elderly.

An age-associated decline in renal function has been well documented although the extent of impairment of renal function will vary significantly among individuals. It is highly desirable to determine creatinine clearance and plasma drug levels when establishing or adjusting dosage levels of drugs that are primarily excreted by the kidneys (eg, digoxin, aminoglycosides) or whose active metabolites are excreted via the kidneys (eg, diazepam, flurazepam). The importance of having such data is underscored when other drugs that can interact through renal (or other) mechanisms are administered concurrently.

MINIMIZING THE RISK
OF DRUG INTERACTION

In most cases, two drugs that are known to interact can be administered concurrently as long as adequate precautions are taken (eg, closer monitoring of therapy, dosage adjustments to compensate for the altered response). Although there are situations where the use of one drug is usually contraindicated while another is being given, such combinations are not likely to be employed frequently and there may be exceptions to the contraindication under certain circumstances. In those situations, though, where another agent with similar therapeutic properties and a lesser risk of interacting could be used, such a course of action would be preferable.

RESPONSIBILITY OF THE HEALTH PROFESSIONAL

The reduction of the risk of drug interactions is a challenge that embraces a number of considerations. Although they could be applied to drug therapy in general, the following principles are offered as guidelines for health professionals having the responsibility for the decisions regarding the selection and monitoring of the therapeutic regimen.

(1) Identify the patient risk factors. The influence of age on the processes of absorption, distribution, metabolism, and excretion have already been noted and, therefore, the age of this patient population must, itself, be viewed as a risk factor. In addition, many of these patients have medical problems associated with impairment of hepatic or renal function, as well as other disorders, which may significantly affect drug action and further increase the risk of interaction. Dietary habits, smoking, and problems like alcoholism will also influence the effect of certain drugs and should be considered during the initial patient interview.

(2) Take a thorough drug history. An accurate and complete record of both the prescription and nonprescription medications a patient is taking must be obtained prior to changing the therapeutic regimen. Numerous interactions have resulted from a lack of awareness of prescription medications prescribed by another physician, or nonprescription medications the patient did not consider important enough to mention.

(3) Maintain complete and current patient medication records. By maintaining patient medication records, the pharmacist is often in a position to

detect potential problems and initiate the necessary steps to minimize or avoid them.

(4) Be knowledgeable about all the drugs being utilized. The knowledge of the properties and the primary and secondary pharmacologic actions of each of the agents used, or being considered for use, is essential if the interaction potential is to be accurately assessed. Therapeutic alternatives that are less likely to interact should be considered.

(5) Keep the potential for interactions in perspective. The extensive publicity that certain drug interactions have received may give the impression that these problems are well identified and can be easily minimized or avoided. Although this may be true in certain circumstances, a careful analysis of the literature reveals that some of the information is conflicting, incomplete, and misleading.

The use of some of this information has, in some circumstances, led to an undue degree of alarm, characterized by some observers as "drug interaction hysteria" or a "drug interaction anxiety syndrome." Caution is needed, therefore, in evaluating and using the information available because by misusing information or by overreacting to a possible problem, a more difficult situation might result than would have occurred if nothing were done. The importance of exercising the appropriate clinical perspective is essential if optimal therapy is to be achieved.

(6) Avoid complex therapeutic regimens where possible. The number of medications utilized should be kept to a minimum. In addition, the use of medications or dosage regimens that permit less-frequent administration may help avoid interactions that result from an alteration of absorption (eg, when a drug is administered in close proximity to meals).

(7) Use smaller doses. The elderly are more sensitive to the actions of many therapeutic agents, and lower dosages are indicated. In addition to reducing the risk of adverse reactions with such agents, the potential for interaction will also be decreased.

(8) Educate the patient. Patients often know little about their illnesses, let alone the benefits and problems that could result from drug therapy. Individuals who are aware of, and understand, this information can be expected to be in greater compliance with the instructions for administering medications and more attentive to the development of symptoms that could be early indicators of drug-related problems. Patients should be encouraged to ask questions about their therapy and to report any excessive or unexpected responses. There should be no uncertainty on the part of the patient as to the manner in which medications should be used to achieve optimum effectiveness and safety.

(9) Therapy should be frequently monitored. The risk of drug-related problems in the elderly warrants close monitoring, not only for the possible occurrence of drug interactions but also for adverse effects occurring with individual agents and noncompliance. Any change in patient behavior should

be suspected as being drug-related until that possibility is excluded. It must be recognized that the symptoms resulting from interactions of the drugs most commonly prescribed in the elderly (eg, psychotropic, cardiovascular, and analgesic drugs) are the same ones that are typically associated with the aging process. Too often, symptoms such as drowsiness, confusion, forgetfulness, anxiety, and anorexia are quickly attributed to "old age" when in fact they are drug-induced and can be prevented through dosage adjustment or modification of the therapeutic regimen.

(10) Therapy must be individualized. Although the development of a therapeutic regimen that meets the specific needs of individual patients is inherent in many of the above guidelines, the importance of this consideration cannot be too strongly emphasized. Wide variations in the response of patients to the same dose of certain individual drugs is well recognized; when recognition is taken of the difficulty in predicting the response of many therapeutic agents when they are given alone, the challenge and limitations in endeavoring to anticipate the response with a multiple drug regimen become apparent. Therefore, priority should be assigned to the needs and clinical response of the individual patient, rather than usual dosage recommendations and standard treatment and monitoring guidelines.

RESPONSIBILITY OF THE PATIENT AND/OR HIS/HER FAMILY

The best efforts of the health professionals involved in the patient's care will fall short of the desired goals unless the patient and/or his/her family participates in, understands, and complies with the decisions regarding the therapeutic regimen. In many situations, the patient will be in a position to fully assume this responsibility, whereas in other circumstances the patient's illnesses may be incapacitating and he or she will have to depend on the assistance of members of the family with respect to the use of medication.

The following guidelines apply to the responsibility of the patient and family and, if observed, should minimize the risk of drug interactions and other drug-related problems.

(1) Discuss the illness(es) and the prescribed medication with the physician. A patient should be knowledgeable about the characteristics of the illness that has been diagnosed as well as the benefits and limitations of medications that have been prescribed.

(2) Select a pharmacy/pharmacist that provides comprehensive professional services. The pharmacy/pharmacist should be selected with the same care with which one selects a physician. Patient medication records should be maintained and the pharmacist should advise the patient regarding the use of medications being dispensed and also be readily available at other times to respond to questions from the patient.

(3) Understand the actions and use of each medication. Patients should know: (a) the name of the prescribed medication, (b) the use and expected actions, (c) the route by which it is administered and any special directions for administration, (d) the specific dosage and the times of the day at which the medication is to be administered, (e) the precautions to be observed during administration (eg, administration with respect to meals), (f) the common side effects that may be encountered, (g) the potential drug-drug and drug-nutrient interactions, (h) the manner in which the medication is to be stored, (i) the expected duration of the therapy and prescription refill information, and (j) considerations regarding monitoring of the therapy.

(4) Ask questions. There should be no uncertainty or basis for misunderstanding with respect to the medication(s) to be used. If there is a question, the physician or pharmacist should be consulted.

(5) Purchase nonprescription medications in the pharmacy. To reduce the risk of drug interactions, nonprescription medications should be purchased in the same pharmacy in which prescription medications are obtained. The use of any nonprescription drug should be discussed with the pharmacist or physician, even if it is purchased elsewhere.

(6) Administer medications in the recommended dosages at the intended times. Any departure from the recommended dosage regimens may increase the possibility that the therapy will be inadequate or that drug-related problems will occur.

(7) Report any effects that may be drug-related to the physician or pharmacist. It is important that drug-related responses be reported promptly to the physician or pharmacist. This is appropriate even for those side effects that might be anticipated, and about which the patient has been cautioned, as an adjustment in dosage may be indicated or there may be steps that can be taken to minimize the extent of the response. It is also possible that the intended beneficial effects of the prescribed medications will not be achieved within the expected time period or that the symptoms of the illness being treated will worsen. Such circumstances should be brought to the physician's attention as the therapeutic regimen may need to be changed.

It is clearly apparent that the patient and/or his/her family are vital members of the team that is responsible for his/her health care. The most accurate diagnosis can be made and the best treatment regimen selected; however, if the patient does not assume the necessary responsibilities, the efforts in his or her behalf will be compromised. Therefore, if the optimal benefits of therapy are to be achieved, with minimal risk, participants must be diligent in observing their individual responsibilities.

Chapter 19

CHANGES IN PHARMACODYNAMIC SENSITIVITY TO DRUGS WITH AGING

B. Robert Meyer, MD

The increased sensitivity of the elderly to a variety of drugs is well established. A great deal of time and effort has gone into the elaboration and clarification of the potential pharmacokinetic changes associated with aging.[1] In contrast, pharmacodynamic changes associated with aging have received relatively little attention. This is due in part to the difficulty in quantifying and systematically studying this phenomonon and also in part to the fact that one cannot definitively demonstrate pharmacodynamic changes until one has effectively ruled out or controlled for the occurrence of pharmacokinetic ones. Despite this fact, there are now several well established examples of pharmacodynamic changes in sensitivity to drugs associated with aging.

BENZODIAZEPINES

Reidenberg et al investigated the dose and serum concentration of diazepam necessary to establish an adequate level of sedation in elderly and young individuals about to undergo elective cardioversion.[2] When compared to young individuals, elderly individuals had lower serum levels of diazepam at identical levels of sedation (Figure 19.1). These results have been confirmed in a similar trial of diazepam dosage in patients undergoing gastrointestinal endoscopy.[3] Castleden et al performed a study of pharmacodynamic sensitivity to the benzodiazepine nitrazepam.[4] They measured psychomotor performance in elderly and young individuals before and after a single dose of 10 mg of oral nitrazepam. They were unable to document pharmacokinetic differences between the young and old subjects but were able to demonstrate that the elderly individuals had significant impairment to psychomotor performance for a period between 36 and 60 hr after the administration of this dose. Young individuals showed no such impairment of function (Figure 19.2).

These studies effectively demonstrate the occurrence of pharmacodynamic sensitivity to the benzodiazepines in the elderly.

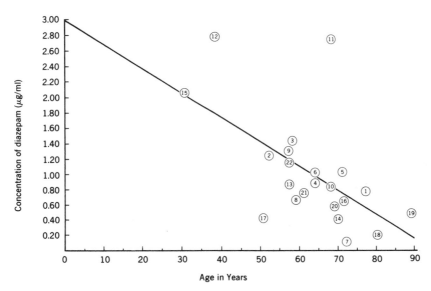

Figure 19.1. Relationship between age and serum diazepam concentration that causes failure to respond to vocal but not painful stimuli.[2]

METOCLOPRAMIDE

Recent investigations of our own have also documented the occurrence of pharmacodynamic sensitivity to metoclopramide in elderly individuals.[5] In the context of a study of metoclopramide control of cis-platinum-induced emesis we measured serum concentrations of metoclopramide 4 hr after beginning a metolcopramide dosing regimen of 2 mg/kg every 2 hr. Elderly individuals in our study had no significant differences in their serum metoclopramide concentrations as compared to younger individuals. However, they appeared to have greater benefit from metoclopramide, and had significantly reduced numbers of emetic episodes in response to identical doses of cis-platinum (Figure 19.3). Because there are no data to suggest changes in platinum sensitivity associated with aging, we interpret these data to provide evidence for pharmacodynamic sensitivity to the effects of metoclopramide.

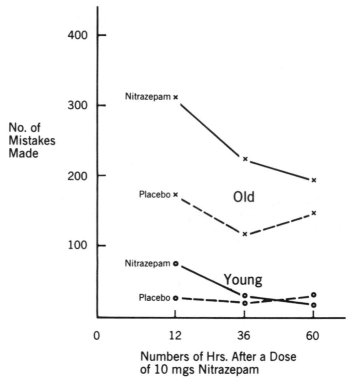

Figure 19.2. Total number of mistakes made in the psychomotor test by each age group after nitrazepam (10 mg) and placebo.[4]

BETA ADRENERGIC AGENTS

Vestal et al have also provided an example of changes in pharmacodynamic sensitivity to drugs in elderly individuals.[6] In contrast to previous studies, they documented a relative decrease in sensitivity associated with the aging process. They administered isoproteranol to a variety of individuals between the ages of 20 and 70 years and calculated the dose of isoproteranol necessary to produce an increase in heart rate of 25 beats/min. Elderly individuals required higher doses than young individuals to produce an identical change in heart rate. Although there are no specific pharmacokinetic data here, this is an acute study and the time between dose and measurement of response was several minutes. It is therefore unlikely that significant pharmacokinetic changes would be present. Subsequently a propranolol infusion was administered to these individuals, propranolol levels were measured, and the Km for propranolol inhibition of isoproteranol effect was calculated. These data demonstrated a clear correlation between age and the Km for propranolol. Like isoproteranol, there is relative propranolol resistance with aging (Figure 19.4).

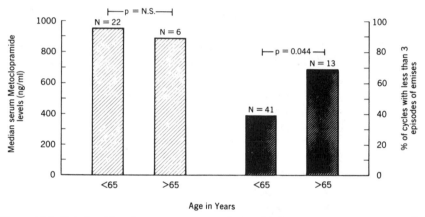

Figure 19.3. Relationship of age to serum metoclopramide levels and episodes of emesis[5]

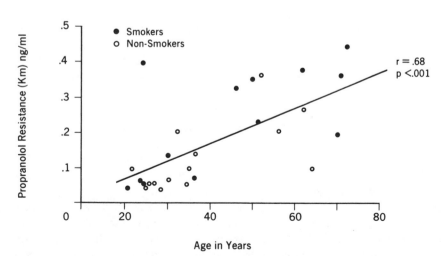

Figure 19.4. Relationship between propranolol resistance and age in smokers and nonsmokers.[6]

REASONS FOR PHARMACODYNAMIC CHANGES

A variety of physiologic changes may be seen as potentially important in the production of altered pharmacodynamic sensitivity. These include alterations in the number of cell receptors for a particular drug, the affinity of those receptors for the drug, and the integrity of the receptor complex as a whole. Postreceptor events, including the effects of the receptor on its second messengers and the subsequent physiologic effects induced in the cell, are also potentially altered in the elderly. Finally, the subsequent effects of the cell on the organ in which it is involved and the changes in the interaction of that organ system with the organism as a whole may also be altered.

In the case of the adrenergic system in the elderly, we have evidence for alterations in virtually all of the components of the pharmacodynamic response. Schocken and Roth[7] and others[8-10] have argued for the occurrence of decreased beta adrenergic receptor concentrations during adulthood and senescence. Roth was among the first to argue this point, presenting data to suggest a substantial decrease in the number of beta-adrenergic receptors in the lymphocytes of elderly individuals. Work by other investigators has failed to confirm this fact; and, the data of Vestal et al, presented earlier in this paper, are most amenable to a different interpretation.[6] They do not suggest changes in hormone receptor number, but are most compatible with a change in beta-receptor sensitivity to agonist and antagonist agents. Other investigators have supported this finding by demonstrating a decrease in lymphocyte adenylate cyclase response to beta-adrenergic agents such as isoproteranol.[11] In the work of Dillon et al, the dose response curve for isoproteranol-induced cyclic AMP production shifted rightwards and downwards with a decrease in the maximal response.[12] This is most compatible with a change in receptor number.

If we move beyond these receptor and immediate postreceptor events, and attempt to see how changes in adrenergic function such as these effect the organism as a whole, we must consider several other concomitant physiologic changes in the elderly. There is evidence for significant changes in the parasympathetic nervous system associated with aging.[13] Sinus arrhythmia, a well described phenomenon in young individuals, and chiefly controlled by vagal activity, is markedly diminished or entirely absent in the elderly population.[14] Similarly, heart rate response to standing, which reflects vagal activity rather more than adrenergic, is also considerably diminished in many elderly individuals.[15,16] Gribbin et al have shown that both normotensive and hypertensive individuals have a significant decrement in baroreflex activity associated with aging.[17] Maintenance of fluid and electrolyte equilibrium, which is critical to the maintenance of normal cardiovascular status is also impaired in the elderly. The relative inability of elderly individuals to concentrate urine and to decrease urinary sodium excretion is well established.[18] All of these factors (1) changes in receptor sensitivity, (2) decreased baroreflex sensitivity, (3) changes in vagal activity or vagal responsiveness, and (4) diminished ability to maintain fluid and electrolyte homeostasis contribute to overall response to adrenergic agents in the elderly.

In contrast to the adrenergic system, in the dopaminergic system there is clear evidence of different sorts of alterations with age. A wide variety of studies have suggested that dopamine receptors in the corpus striatum decline with aging.[19,20] There is a decline in dopamine neurotransmitter production and diminished responsiveness of this system to exogenous dopamine administration.[21] In young rats, the administration of a dopamine-blocking agent tends to induce a secondary increase in dopamine receptors. In older rats no such change is observed.[22] In our study of elderly individuals receiving metoclopramide, the increased sensitivity to metoclopramide may be a function of these changes, with decreased receptor numbers leading to increased sensitivity to inhibitory agents.

In the case of GABA receptors and the benzodiazepines, there is as yet no clear answer. Contradictory evidence in the literature would suggest both the presence and absence of changes in receptor number, as well as potential occurrence of alterations in receptor affinity and responsiveness.[23,24]

CONCLUSIONS

When we first began to investigate pharmacokinetic changes associated with aging, it was hoped that simple and easily definable changes associated with the aging process would allow us to make simple and easily predictable changes in our drug dosing recommendations for the elderly. As the subject has been investigated, the variety of changes, or lack thereof, seen with the aging process has become appreciated. Similarly, there does not appear to be a single simple answer to the question of mechanisms for pharmacodynamic sensitivity associated with aging. Instead there appears to be a variety of subtle changes in various steps in the pharmacodynamic response, which in their aggregate produce the observed phenomenon of altered sensitivity. Furthermore, the mechanisms for altered sensitivity appear to vary for each drug that we consider.

Elderly individuals are sensitive to a variety of interventions in their physiologic homeostasis. They have diminished ability to adapt to changes in ambient temperature,[13,25,26] decreased ability to autoregulate cerebral blood flow in response to hypoxia,[27] and decreased ability to respond to illness or trauma.[28] In each instance, close investigation reveals that the altered responsiveness of the elderly is not the result of an isolated alteration in their physiologic function but the result of a complex change in physiologic homeostasis associated with aging. The occurrence of orthostatic hypotension in the elderly population is well documented. In one study, some 24% of elderly individuals had a greater than 20 mm Hg drop in systolic blood pressure when assuming a standing position. A full 9% of this population had a 30 mm Hg or greater drop in blood pressure, and 5% of this population had a 40 mm Hg or greater decline in blood pressure.[29] This abnormality in the maintenance of cardiovascular homeostasis reflects many of the changes we have elaborated earlier. It reflects a decrease in baroreflex sensitivity, coupled with changes in a baseline level of circulating catecholamines, changes in sensitivity of receptors to these catecholamines, changes in vascular tissue elasticity and responsiveness, changes in fluid homeostasis and maintenance of intravascular volume, and increased peripheral pooling in venous varicosities.[30]

All of these wide variety of stimuli require a fairly complex series of adaptive physiologic changes in an attempt to maintain bodily homeostasis. The administration of a pharmacologic agent to an elderly individual is a similar intervention whose net effect is the result of a complex series of physiologic responses. The sensitivity of the elderly individual to these pharmacologic manipulations, like their sensitivity to the orthostatic changes in position, will be the result of a complex summary of a variety of physiologic changes. When we look closely at any of the drugs to which the elderly have a pharmacodynamic sensitivity, we will have to evaluate a variety of factors such as those elaborated here to adequately assess the reasons for their altered sensitivity.

REFERENCES

1. Greenblatt DJ, Sellers EM, Shader RI: Drug disposition in old age. *N Engl J Med* 1982; 306:1081–1088.

2. Reidenberg MM, Levy M, Warner H, et al: Relationship between diazepam dose, plasma level, age, and central nervous system depression. *Clin Pharm Ther* 1978; 23:371–374.

3. Giles HG, Macleod SM, Wright JR, et al: Influence of age and previous use on diazepam dosage required for endoscopy. *Can Med Assoc J* 1978; 118:513–514.

4. Castleden CM, George CF, Marcer D, et al: Increased sensitivity to nitrazepam in old age. *Br Med J* 1977; 1:10–12.

5. Meyer BR, Lewin M, Pasmantier M, et al: Optimizing metoclopramide control of cis-platin-induced emesis. *Ann Inter Med* 1984; 100:393–395.

6. Vestal RE, Wood AJJ, Shand DG: Reduced beta adrenoreceptor sensitivity in the elderly. *Clin Pharmacol Ther* 1979; 26:181–186.

7. Schocken DD, Roth GS: Reduced beta andrenergic receptor concentrations in aging man. *Nature* 1977; 267:856–858.

8. Guidicelli Y, Perquery R: Beta-adrenergic receptors and catecholamine sensitive adenylate cyclase in rat fat cell membranes: Influence of growth, cell size, and aging. *Eur J Biochem* 1978; 90:413–419.

9. Byland DM, Tellex-Inon MT, Hollenberg MD: Age-related parallel decline in beta-adrenergic receptors, adenylate cyclase, and phosphodiesterase activity in rat erythrocyte membranes. *Life Sci* 1977; 21:403–407.

10. Freilich JS, Weiss B: Altered adaptive capacity of brain catecholaminergic receptors during aging, in Samuel D, et al (eds): *Aging of the Brain*. New York, Raven Press, 1983, pp 277–300.

11. Krall JF, Connelly M, Weisbart R, et al: Age-related elevation of plasma catecholamine concentration and reduced responsiveness of lymphocyte adenylate cyclase. *J Clin Endoc Metab* 1981; 52:863–867.

12. Dillon N, Chung S, Kelly J, et al: Age and beta adrenoceptor-mediated function. *Clin Pharmacol Ther* 1980; 27:769–772.

13. Collins KJ: Autonomic failure and the elderly, in Bannister R (ed): *Autonomic Failure*. Oxford, Oxford University Press, 1983, pp 489–507.

14. Smith SE, Smith SA: Heart rate variability in healthy subjects measured with a bedside computer-based technique. *Clin Sci* 1981; 61:379–383.

15. Ewing DJ, Campbell IW, Murray A, et al: Immediate heart rate response to standing: simple test for autonomic neuropathy in diabetes. *Br Med J* 1978; 1:145–147.

16. Collin KJ, James NH, Oliver DJ: Functional changes in autonomic nervous responses with aging. *Age Aging* 1980; 9:17–24.

17. Gribbin B, Pickering TG, Sleight P, et al: Effect of age and high blood pressure on baroreflex sensitivity in man. *Circ Res* 1971: 29:424–431.

18. Epstein M, Hollenberg NK: Age as a determinant of renal sodium conservation in normal men. *J Lab Clin Med* 1976: 87:411.

19. Makman NH, Ahn HS, Thal LJ, et al: Aging and monoamine receptors in brain. *Fed Proc* 1979: 38:1922–1926.

20. Joseph JA, Roth GS: Age-related alterations in dopaminergic mechanisms, in Samuel D, et al (eds): *Aging of the Brain*. New York, Raven Press, 1983, pp 245–256.

21. Roth G: Altered mechanisms of opiate and dopaminergic action during aging, in Giacobini E, et al (eds): *The Aging Brain: Cellular and Molecular Mechanisms of Aging in the Nervous System*. New York, Raven Press, 1982, pp 203–209.

22. Trabucchi M, Spano PF, Govoni S, et al: Dopaminergic function during aging in rat brain, in Giacobini E, et al (eds): *The Aging Brain: Cellular and Molecular Mechanisms of Aging in the Nervous System*. New York, Raven Press, 1982, pp 195–201.

23. Govoni S, Memo M, Saiani L: Impairment of brain transmitter neuroreceptors in aged rats. *Mech Aging Dev* 1980; 12:39–46.

24. Kendall DA, Strong R, Enna SJ: Modifications in rat brain GABA receptor binding as a function of age, in Giacobini E, et al (eds): *The Aging Brain: Cellular and Molecular Mechanisms of Aging in the Nervous System*. New York, Raven Press, 1982, pp 211–221.

25. Collins KJ, Easton JC, Exton-Smith AN: Shivering thermogenesis and vasomotor responses with convective cooling in the elderly. *J Physiol Lond* 1981; 320:76.

26. Foster KG, Ellis FP, Dur C, et al: Sweat responses in the aged. *Age Aging* 1976; 5:91-101.

27. Wollner L, McCarthy ST, Soper NDW, Macy DJ: Failure of cerebral auto-regulation as a cause of brain dysfunction in the elderly. *Br Med J* 1979; 1:1117-1118.

28. Hogue CC: Injury in late life, Part I Epidemiology. *J Am Ger Soc* 1982; 30:183.

29. Caird FI, Andrews GR, Kennedy RD: Effect of position on blood pressure in the elderly. *Br Heart J* 1973; 35:527-530.

30. Anonymous: Posture, pressure, and advancing years. *Lancet* 1983; 2:87.

Chapter 20

PHARMACOKINETIC RISK FACTORS IN THE ELDERLY

David J. Greenblatt, MD,
Darrell R. Abernethy, MD, PhD,
and Richard I. Shader, MD

For many drugs used in clinical practice, the steady state concentration in blood, serum, or plasma is proportional to the steady state concentration at the receptor site, and that concentration is a major determinant of clinical outcome. When the concentration is in the proper therapeutic range, we have therapeutically efficacious drug therapy. When the concentration is too high, we have potential toxicity; when the concentration is too low, we have therapeutic ineffectiveness.

One major objective of the art or science of drug therapy is to achieve and maintain therapeutic steady state concentrations (Css). The two principal determinants of Css are as follows:

$$Css = \frac{Dosing\ Rate}{Clearance.}$$

In the numerator is dosing rate; in the denominator is clearance. The numerator is a health care professional-controlled variable: dosing rate, or the rate at which the drug is administered. The health care professional chooses the dosing rate and therefore has control over that determinant of the steady state concentration.

The authors are grateful for the collaboration and assistance of Hermann R. Ochs, Marcia K. Divoll, and Jerald S. Harmatz. This study was supported in part by Grants MH-34223 and AM-MH-32050 for the United States Public Health Service.

In the denominator is clearance, which is entirely a biologically controlled variable over which health care professionals have no control. Clearance has units of volume divided by time, and reflects that given individual's capacity to biotransform, excrete, or remove that particular drug. Clearance can be conceptualized as the hypothetical total amount of blood or plasma from which the substance is completely removed per unit time.

With regard to drug therapy in the elderly, we are principally concerned about the elevation of steady state concentration that may occur as a result of reduced drug clearance. That in turn may lead to unexpected or unwanted drug toxicity, unless the health care professional intervenes to appropriately change the dosing rate. The discipline of pharmacogeriatrics is the study of drug effects in the elderly, and the alterations of drug absorption, distribution, and clearance that may occur in the aging population.

Pharmacogeriatrics is of importance for two reasons. First, it provides clinical information to improve drug therapy in the elderly. If we can predict, understand, and anticipate changes in drug clearance that are associated with old age, then we should be in a position to alter dosing rates to maintain steady state concentrations in the therapeutic range, and prevent excessively high drug concentrations and potential drug toxicity. Second, pharmacogeriatrics contributes to our general understanding of mechanisms controlling the fate of foreign chemicals.

CLEARANCE, VOLUME OF DISTRIBUTION, AND HALF-LIFE

Research over the years has taught the importance of identifying the correct endpoint in studies of drug metabolism in old age.[1,2] Clearance is an independent variable, quantitating a given person's capacity to remove a given foreign chemical. Clearance is accomplished by clearing organs, and the two principal clearing organs responsible for removal of foreign chemicals are the kidney and the liver. Not surprisingly, the clearance of a foreign chemical cannot exceed the delivery of blood to the clearing organs.

Elimination half-life, on the other hand, is a potentially misleading variable, because it is related directly to volume of distribution (Vd) and inversely to clearance. If Vd does not change, half-life will inversely reflect changes in clearance. In the elderly, however, Vd may change because body habitus has changed, thereby altering the profile of drug distribution to various tissues.

Thus half-life is a dependent variable, related to two biologically distinct independent variables. Clearance is the capacity of the organism to remove that particular compound, whereas Vd reflects the profile or pattern of drug distribution to various tissues in the body. If we are studying a situation in which Vd is relatively constant, then half-life will inversely reflect clearance.

On the other hand, in pharmacogeriatrics, changes in drug distribution may be at least as important as changes in clearance, so that clearance and Vd can change concurrently in the same direction or in different directions, thereby confounding the meaning of half-life.[3]

For example, consider two drugs of different characteristics, studied in a series of male volunteers ranging in age from 20 to 80 years. If we look at the relatively water-soluble compound antipyrine, then we find a highly significant decline in antipyrine Vd relative to total weight, reflecting the decrease in lean mass relative to total weight that occurs with age (Figure 20.1).

On the other hand, if we look at the highly lipid-soluble drug diazepam in the same individuals, Vd increases significantly in association with age (Figure 20.1). Thus, the shift away from lean mass towards adipose tissue that occurs as a function of age may change the volume of distribution of drugs, depending on whether they are water soluble or lipid soluble. This in turn can change half-lives of drugs, thereby emphasizing the need to study clearance rather than only elimination half-life.

ROUTES OF DRUG CLEARANCE

The two principal routes responsible for eliminating foreign chemicals are excretion by the kidney or biotransformation by the liver. In the case of the kidney, the change in its function with age is relatively predictable. A number of studies demonstrate significant reductions in creatinine clearance in association with the aging process, even in the absence of any detectable evidence of overt renal disease.[4-6] This has implications for those few drugs whose primary route of clearance is intact excretion by the kidney. These include, for example, digoxin, lithium, cimetidine, procainamide, and the aminoglycoside antibiotics.

When one is prescribing those renally cleared drugs for the elderly, a need for reduction in dosage must be anticipated. How much reduction in dosage is needed depends on that particular individual's precise value of creatinine clearance. Although we can find a fairly predictable decline in creatinine clearance with age on the average, we cannot predict creatinine clearance in a particular individual without measuring it.[5] Serum creatinine alone is a potentially misleading index of renal function because serum creatinine reflects not only creatinine clearance but also creatinine production, which in turn reflects muscle mass and muscle turnover. One can have a significant and clinically important decline in creatinine clearance with very little change in serum creatinine. Clinical laboratories are of little help with this interpretation.

The liver is a much more complicated organ, since it behaves almost as if it were two organs — one performing oxidation and the other performing conjugation. In reality, these two classes of reactions occur side-by-side in

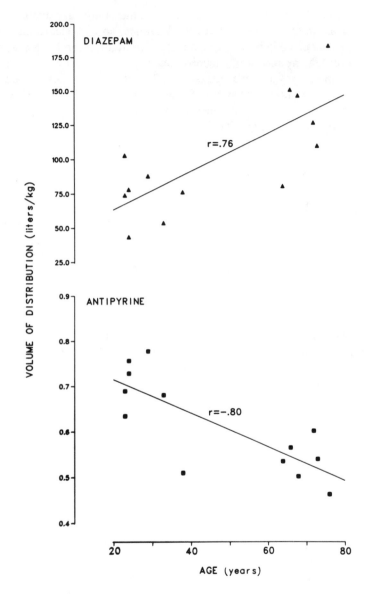

Figure 20.1. Relation of age to Vd for antipyrine and diazepam among 13 healthy male volunteers who received single intravenous doses of both drugs on two occasions. Solid lines were determined by linear regression analysis. Values of diazepam Vd were corrected for protein binding, yielding unsound Vd. See References 7 and 16 for details of the studies. (Reprinted from Reference 1, with permission)

the same hepatocyte, but the mechanisms of control are very different. The principal oxidative reactions are hydroxylation and N-dealkylation. The principal conjugative reactions are glucuronide conjugation and sulfate conjugation. They are fundamentally different reactions, and they are influenced differently by age.

PHARMACOKINETICS OF DRUGS IN THE ELDERLY

For oxidized drugs such as antipyrine, whose total clearance is considerably less than hepatic blood flow, there is a decline in oxidizing capacity associated with the aging process.[7] However, the changes in antipyrine clearance with age are relatively gender-specific, with a far greater decrement in elderly men than in elderly women. For essentially every other low-clearance oxidized compound that we have studied, a similar reduction in oxidizing capacity with age has been observed, usually more so in men that in women.[8-16] Furthermore, the antipyrine clearance test appears to identify these individuals with impaired capacity to oxidize other drugs where clearance is much less than hepatic blood flow.[7,8] In the case of high-clearance oxidized drugs, things may be more complicated, since hepatic blood flow as well as enzyme activity may influence clearance.[17]

With regard to conjugated compounds, on the other hand, conjugating capacity is relatively uninfluenced by age. We have studied a number of drugs that are biotransformed by conjugation including oxazepam, lorazepam, temazepam, and acetaminophen. For these compounds, clearance is minimally if at all influenced by age.[18-22]

We conclude that old age is associated with impaired drug oxidation, which in some cases is relatively gender-specific. In general, the elderly may be at risk of excessive drug accumulation for compounds that are biotransformed by oxidation. This appears to be a reasonably replicable pharmacokinetic risk factor. Drug conjugation, on the other hand, is far less, if at all, influenced by age. For conjugated drugs, pharmacokinetics per se is not really a risk factor. However, that does not rule out the possibility of pharmacodynamic risk factors independent of pharmacokinetics.

COMMENT

The sources of variance influencing drug metabolizing capacity are numerous. Age is one of them, but there are many others. In most studies, age accounts for a significant amount of variance but still is not the principal determinant of variance. A large fraction of variance remains unexplained.

REFERENCES

1. Greenblatt DJ, Sellers EM, Shader RI: Drug disposition on old age. *N Eng J Med* 1982; 306:1081-1088.

2. Vestal RE: Drug use in the elderly. *Drugs* 1978; 16:358-382.

3. Abernethy DR, Greenblatt DJ: Pharmacokinetics of drugs in obesity. *Clin Pharmacokinet* 1982; 7:108-124.

4. Rowe JW, Andres R, Tobin JD, et al: The effects of age on creatinine clearance in man. *J Gerontol* 1976; 31:155-163.

5. Ochs HR, Greenblatt DJ, Harmatz JS, et al: Clinical implications of serum digoxin concentrations. *Klin Wochenschr* 1981; 59:501-507.

6. Friedman SA, Raizner AE, Rosen H, et al: Functional defects in the aging kidney. *Ann Inter Med* 1972; 76:41-45.

7. Greenblatt DJ, Divoll M, Abernethy DR, et al: Antipyrine kinetics in the elderly: Prediction of age-related changes in benzodiazepine oxidizing capacity. *J Pharmacol Exp Ther* 1982; 220:120-126.

8. Greenblatt DJ, Divoll M, Abernethy DR, et al: Alprazolam kinetics in the elderly: Relation to antipyrine disposition. *Arch Gen Psychiatry* 1983; 40:287-290.

9. Greenblatt DJ, Divoll M, Puri SK, et al: Reduced single-dose clearance of clobazam in elderly men predicts increased multiple-dose accumulation. *Clin Pharmacokinet* 1983; 8:83-94.

10. Divoll M, Greenblatt DJ, Ochs HR, et al: Absolute bioavailability of oral and intramuscular diazepam: Effect of age and sex. *Anesthesia Analgesia* 1983; 62:1-8.

11. Shader RI, Greenblatt DJ, Ciraulo DA, et al: Effect of age and sex on disposition of desmethyldiazepam formed from its precursor clorazepate. *Psychopharmacology* 1981; 75:193-197.

12. Greenblatt DJ, Divoll M, Puri SK, et al: Clobazam kinetics in the elderly. *Br J Clin Pharmacol* 1981; 12:631-636.

13. Greenblatt DJ, Divoll M, Harmatz JS, et al: Kinetics and clinical effects of flurazepam in young and elderly noninsomniacs. *Clin Pharmacol Ther* 1981; 30:475-486.

14. Shader RI, Greenblatt DJ, Harmatz JS, et al: Absorption and disposition of chlordiazepoxide in young and elderly male volunteers. *J Clin Pharmacol* 1977; 17:709-718.

15. Allen MD, Greenblatt DJ, Harmatz JS, et al: Desmethyldiazepam kinetics in the elderly after oral prazepam. *Clin Pharmacol Ther* 1980; 28:196-202.

16. Greenblatt DJ, Allen MD, Harmatz JS, et al: Diazepam disposition determinants. *Clin Pharmacol Ther* 1980; 27:301-312.

17. Greenblatt DJ, Divoll M, Abernethy DR, et al: Reduced clearance of triazolam in old age: Relation to antipyrine oxidizing capacity. *Br J Clin Pharmacol* 1983; 15:303-309.

18. Greenblatt DJ, Allen MD, Locniskar A, et al: Lorazepam kinetics in the elderly. *Clin Pharmacol Ther* 1979; 26:103-113.

19. Divoll M, Greenblatt DJ, Harmatz JS, et al: Effect of age and gender on disposition of temazepam. *J Pharm Sci* 1981; 70:1104-1107.

20. Ochs HR, Greenblatt DJ, Otten H: Disposition of oxazepam in relation to age, sex, and cigarette smoking. *Klin Wochenschr* 1981; 59:899-903.

21. Greenblatt DJ, Divoll M, Harmatz JS, et al: Oxazepam kinetics: Effects of age and sex. *J Pharmacol Exp Ther* 1980; 215:86-91.

22. Divoll M, Abernethy DR, Ameer B, et al: Acetaminophen kinetics in the elderly. *Clin Pharmacol Ther* 1982; 31:151-156.

Chapter 21

RISK FACTORS IN GERIATRIC DRUG USE: BIOBEHAVIORAL ISSUES

Robert Straus, PhD

Most studies of risk factors for geriatric drug use involve either surveys that describe and interpret the behavior of individuals who prescribe and use drugs or investigations into the biological processes that occur when drugs are administered to human beings. This chapter will discuss the need for a conceptual approach that recognizes and addresses the fundamental interface of these biological and behavioral phenomena. There are several compelling reasons why it is important to consider biological and behavioral factors within a common frame of reference. First and most obvious is the fact that, whereas the actions of drugs on the body involve biological processes, the actions that determine what drugs are used by whom, how, when, and under what circumstances are clearly behavioral.

Second, there is evidence of considerable biological variability in the ways in which human beings respond to drugs, and it has been found that such variability increases with advancing age. Yet, most drug use behavior is in accordance with prescribing patterns and utilizing customs that neither recognize nor respect biological variability.

Third, we are experiencing rapid changes in the nature of drugs and their potential for benefit and harm and also changes in the human conditions for which drugs are used. These include demographic and lifestyle characteristics as well as the nature, prevalence, and distribution of diseases. Yet the beliefs and practices that constitute drug prescribing and using behavior are changing more slowly. Thus, a fairly large gap exists between biological knowledge about drugs and how they affect people and the beliefs on which prescribing and utilizing practices are based.

Fourth, risks associated with use of medications are inseparable from numerous related aspects of human behavior, including nutrition practices;

the uses of alcohol, tobacco, and caffeine; and the use of a variety of nonmedical substances. They are also inseparable from such important aspects of human behavior as work, sex, and recreation.

COMPONENTS OF A BIOBEHAVIORAL CONCEPTUAL APPROACH

From a conceptual viewpoint, I would like to suggest that all behavior, no matter how insignificant or obscure, involves a fundamental interaction among factors that are biological, psychological, social, cultural, environmental, and temporal. Within each of these six components of behavior, specific characteristics provide potentialities and impose limitations on behavior that affect the interface with other components.

Biological characteristics include the structure, the function, and the chemistry of the human body. For many of these characteristics, there are ranges of potential development that are genetically determined. But, within genetically determined ranges of biological potential, the actual characteristics of the individual are determined by behavioral factors. For example, if we assume that each individual is born with fixed ranges of potential growth, the actual achieved growth within this range will be determined by experiential factors that include nutritional behavior. If we assume genetically determined ranges of potential strength, the actual strength attained will depend upon such behavioral factors as nutrition and the extent to which the musculoskeletal system is exercised. If we assume a potential range of memory capacity, the actual memory capacity achieved will depend upon practice and utilization of memory. In a similar way, we can assume potential ranges of responses to a particular drug. Some people may display toxic sensitivity at any time that they are exposed to the drug. Others may only become sensitive when they are exposed at a particular dosage level. Others may develop sensitivity only when a particular dosage level is experienced on a cumulative basis. Others may only develop sensitivity when they are fatigued or suffering from a viral infection or when the drug interacts with a particular food or alcohol or another drug. Others may experience the sensitivity only when they have reached a particular stage of development in the aging process.

There is considerable current research interest in the alcohol field, and also in research on other drugs, that is focusing on alternative metabolic pathways. Such a pathway for alcohol, the microsomal ethanol oxidizing system (MEOS), has been identified. It is hypothesized that the activation of this and possible other metabolic pathways involves a combination of a genetically determined capability for activating the pathway and a behaviorally experienced cumulative exposure to the relevant substance (ethanol). Some individuals may have no capacity for an alternative pathway irrespective of their drinking behavior. Some may activate the pathway only with prolonged heavy use, others may activate the pathway with moderate use, and some may activate the pathway with any use. Similar hypotheses may help explain synergistic reactions that occur in some individuals but not in others when certain drugs are used simultaneously.

Relationships between biological functioning and psychological factors have long been recognized by those concerned with psychosomatic medicine. More recently, the fields of behavioral medicine, environmental and occupational medicine, behavioral immunology, and behavioral pharmacology have broadened our perceptions of the scope of relevant biobehavioral factors.

Relevant psychological characteristics in a biobehavioral concept include such factors as personality traits, moods, learning, intelligence, memory, pain and stress thresholds, assorted brain functions, and the psychological processes involved in positive and negative reinforcement and dependency. All of these psychological characteristics are subject to the impact of drug use and, in turn, are significant determinants of individual drug utilization. Many drugs act directly on the central nervous system and alter both brain functions and moods. Yet it is important to recognize that the psychological concomitants of drug use are by no means restricted to mood-modifying drugs. Studies of the placebo effect illustrate how psychological processes can influence the perceived impact of a wide variety of drugs.

Social factors involved in drug utilization include the varied roles that individuals fill in society with respect to their families, their work, their community; the groups and organizations that individuals belong to and identify with; and the combination of social and economic factors that tend to determine beliefs and values, define social status, and prescribe social behavior. It is with social groups that drug-use customs and expectations are learned and reinforced. Social support systems have been found to be highly significant in relation to drug-use adherence or compliance. Many individuals with chronic disabling diseases are able to function effectively within their social roles and to fulfill social expectations only because of the medications that they are using. At the same time, the adverse effects of medications can interface with certain roles as, for example, when drugs that provide sedation interface with tasks that require uncompromised brain function. With aging, there are changes in the social roles that individuals are filling and in their family and other group affiliations that are clearly affected by and, in turn, can affect drug utilization.

The cultural components of behavior include both material and normative factors. Material culture includes the systems of invention, discovery, manufacture, and distribution that provide drugs. They include the economic factors of drug production and utilization, factors of cost and buying power, and factors of rapidly changing technology. Currently, developing processes for automatically determining desirable dosage and for facilitating the appropriate self-administration of drugs offer great promise for reducing drug-use risks in our aging population and for creating a more favorable balance between the benefits and adverse outcomes of medication utilization.

The normative aspects of culture include traditions, values, beliefs, customs, and accepted ways of behavior. These comprise powerful determinants of drug utilization. Prescribing patterns of physicians generally are in accordance with established norms and tend to give relatively little attention to individual variability. Marketing practices and advertising tend to create and support drug-use norms.

Environmental factors in drug-use risks include the environmental barriers of space and distance that may make it difficult for individuals, particularly aging individuals, to obtain medical care and similar barriers that have been identified by older people who have been unable to obtain prescribed drugs. There are also environmental factors associated with the safe storage of drugs. For example, most people use bathroom medicine cabinets or kitchen shelves where drugs are particularly vulnerable to moisture and steam. Appropriate environmental arrangements can facilitate the convenient and effective use of drugs. The interface of environment and drug use is also illustrated by the ways in which drugs can facilitate a handicapped individual's ability to cope with the environment.

Nursing homes constitute a particular kind of environment in which drugs are often used in order to control patients or enhance administrative convenience. More research is needed on variations in drug utilization for patients with similar conditions who are living in institutional settings compared with those who are living in family and community settings.

The variable of time is often overlooked in both biological and behavioral research, and yet it is clearly relevant to several dimensions of drug utilization. Time cycles such as the circadian rhythm, the menstrual cycle, and, indeed, the life cycle have been identified with numerous changes in biological functioning. Yet, despite the evidence that some drugs are utilized by the body at varying rates around the circadian clock, it is only rarely that current prescribing practices take such variability into account. Evidence of significant pharmacokinetic and pharmacodynamic changes that occur in the life cycle has also been relatively slow to influence prescribing practices. Perception of time by individuals is a critical variable that influences adherence and compliance with drug use regimens. The extent to which people are oriented to the past, the present, or the future is also an important variable. It is particularly significant that people who lack future orientation may also lack appreciation of the importance of medications, such as hypertension drugs, that are used in the present in order to prevent problems in the future. Time is a significant variable in the prescriber-patient relationship and the failure to use appropriate time may limit the prescriber's knowledge of the patient, the effectiveness of communication with the patient about appropriate drug utilization, and the desirable monitoring of benefits or adverse effects produced by the medication.

CONFLICT BETWEEN BIOLOGICAL VARIABILITY AND NORMS

As new medications are developed with an ever-increasing potential for relieving stress and facilitating recovery, they tend to be more complex. At the same time, they tend to require more precision in their use in order to maximize their benefits and minimize their adverse effects. Recently, new knowledge in genetics, the neurosciences, biochemistry, and pharmacology has brought about an increasing recognition of the variability of responses of different individuals to many medications and other drugs. Not only is there recognition of marked variability of response between individuals, but there is increasing recognition that specific individuals vary in their response to particular drugs under different conditions. As already mentioned, there are variations in response according to biological rhythms such as the circadian cycle, the menstrual cycle, and the life cycle, and there are variations according to conditions such as fatigue, recent illness, nutritional status, and the use of alcohol, tobacco, caffeine, and other drugs.

Yet, despite what has become a fairly well established body of knowledge about variable response to drugs, most prescribing of medications is still based on relatively standardized norms. To be sure, recommended dosages call for smaller amounts for infants and children than for adults. But, beyond "childhood," there is little variation in prescribing norms whether measured by the directions that are suggested by manufacturers or by actual practices as they have been identified in studies of prescribing patterns. If my own recent experience with my dog is at all typical, veterinarians may be ahead of many physicians in recognizing the significance of the circadian cycle and time-related dosage. In prescribing a steroid for my dog, my veterinarian recently gave explicit instructions that the drug should be administered between 7 a.m. and 10 a.m. every other day. This was because early morning is the time of day when a dog's body can be expected to utilize this particular drug most effectively and alternate-day administration would help avoid an adverse effect of the drug on the dog's immune mechanism.

FACTORS OF RAPID CHANGE

We have already alluded to changes in the nature of drugs. As new drugs are being developed, they tend to be more complex, more specific in their action, and, along with great potential for benefit, they carry great risk of harm if they are misused. Also, we are on the threshold of new technology that will enable us automatically to adjust the dosage of some drugs to varying biological need.

Changes in the nature of our population are also occurring rapidly. Specifically, we are becoming a society with more older people, who have more degenerative diseases and who can be expected to use more drugs and to become involved in more complex medication regimens in which they are taking several drugs simultaneously for multiple conditions. Other significant changes include an increasing general faith that medicines will be found that can relieve symptoms and cure disease. This faith is illustrated by the widespread public demand for new drugs that tends to occur whenever they are publicized and often long before there has been very much experience with their use. There is a widespread dependence on medicines on the part of prescribers as well as the general public. More recently, however, there is also a growing awareness of problems of medicine misuse. Episodes such as the tragedies produced by thalidomide and DES have brought about public awareness of the concept (though not the term) of teratology while the epidemic of nonmedicinal drug abuse has made the public somewhat more aware of the dangers of drug dependence including dependence on medicinal drugs. Anecdotal descriptions of harmful consequences of multiple medication interactions have appeared in the public press and have become common when people compare their medical experiences. Together, these events have somewhat tempered what is still a widespread faith in medications.

Another significant change is the relatively recent emphasis on modern preventive medicine and health promotion in which discussions of "health style" identify medicine misuse along with smoking, drinking, sedentary living, and poor diet as major contributing factors to death and disability. The consequences of rapid change are seen in a gap between the potential benefits of modern medicines and the actual benefits experienced by our society. This gap includes inadequate knowledge on the part of prescribers about the drugs they are prescribing and about the patients for whom they are prescribing. The risks associated with inadequate knowledge become great as the population becomes older because people tend to have more illnesses, to use more medications, and more often to use several medications simultaneously. As noted, the significance of individual variability in response to drugs appears to increase as people get older. There is also a large communication gap with respect to information provided to patients by prescribers regarding what medications they are taking, why, when, how, and about problems of drug interaction and adverse effect. Finally, there is a serious failure on the part of most prescribers to monitor the experiences that patients are having with drugs so that they can appropriately ascertain whether benefits are being achieved and whether there are adverse effects.

OTHER RELATED BEHAVIORS

Prescribers of complex medications not only frequently fail to seek adequate information about their patients' medication-using experiences in order to identify histories of sensitivities to particular drugs and take into account other prescriptions and over-the-counter medications that their patients are currently using, but they also tend to neglect seeking information about other substances that can interact with medications and significantly affect their impact. In particular, the alcohol-use histories and practices of patients are often omitted from medical histories. When drugs that can interact with alcohol are prescribed, instructions regarding the consequences of such interactions are often omitted. Similar problems exist with respect to smoking, caffeine use, and nutrition, despite the large and growing body of knowledge regarding the ways in which medications can interact with certain foods, alcohol, and substances like caffeine and tobacco so that their actions are significantly altered. There is also often neglect of the relevance of such basic aspects of behavior as the patients' work, families, responsibilities, sexual activities, life styles, beliefs, and fears or anxieties about their illnesses or medications. Communication about such activities is particularly important when medications are being prescribed that can compromise work, sexual, or interpersonal activities, or can produce anxiety-raising effects.

THE CASE OF HYPERTENSION

In summarizing this discussion of biobehavioral factors in medication risk for the elderly, I will draw examples from a discussion of hypertension.

Hypertension is a widespread condition for which both incidence and prevalence increase with aging. The health risk consequences of hypertension also appear to increase with advancing age with a longer duration of experiencing the cumulative effects of the condition. Hypertension is believed to be caused by several factors. There are ranges of biological vulnerability and there are numerous types of behavior that appear to increase the risk that those who are vulnerable will develop the condition. Some behavioral risks such as the use of too much salt or caffeine or alcohol, being overweight, or lack of exercise convey their own varying dimensions of biological vulnerability. People thus vary in the extent to which different biological and behavioral factors cause hypertension and in the extent to which biological and behavioral intervention can help control the condition.

From the perspective of risks in drug use, all of the several types of medication that are effective in controlling hypertension can produce undesirable effects. Many of these adverse effects are experienced in both biological and behavioral terms. They include distressing neurological symptoms, and profound alteration of mood, along with impairment of cognitive, motor, and sexual functioning. The prescribing norms of some hypertension drugs tend to call for amounts that exceed the dosage necessary to control hypertension in many persons, thus raising, perhaps unnecessarily, the risks and incidence of adverse behavioral effects. Because of the undesirable behavioral consequences that such drugs can produce, many patients do not adhere to their medication regimens.

For older people, in whom the adverse effects of medication can have heightened biological and behavioral consequences, it becomes particularly important that medications be prescribed in forms that will achieve the desired effect with minimum undesirable impact. This requires prescribers who are knowledgeable about the patients for whom they are prescribing, the conditions for which they are prescribing, and the multiple potential effects of the drugs that they are prescribing. It behooves us to cultivate a biobehavioral perspective on the basis of which recognition and consideration of relevant interrelated biological and behavioral factors can become part of the prescribing practice.

PART 8

CLINICAL TESTING OF DRUGS IN THE ELDERLY

Chapter 22

FDA CLINICAL GUIDELINES FOR STUDYING DRUGS IN THE ELDERLY

Robert Temple, MD

Several months ago we at the FDA made available a "discussion paper" on the testing of drugs in the elderly. It was in essence a preproposed guideline. The paper offered a general overall approach to the evaluation of the effects of any drug in the elderly and was based on several premises:

1. The problems of drugs in the elderly are only in part, in perhaps small part, the result of age per se. They are also the result of illness or influences that can occur at any age but may be more common in the elderly.

2. Much of the information needed to use drugs safely in the elderly can be derived both from the elderly and from younger patients such as:

- how the drug is metabolized and excreted and therefore what derangements might influence metabolism or excretion

- the relationship of blood levels of drug to pharmacologic effect (This may be altered in the elderly but this cannot be learned until the nonelderly are well studied.)

- the presence of drug-drug interactions, either pharmacokinetic or pharmacodynamic

- the presence of drug-disease interaction

3. The elderly are so heterogeneous with respect to physiologic processes, other drug use, and concomitant illness that their specific problems can best be identified if a broad range of elderly patients are included in trials and multivariate techniques are used to distinguish the influence of age per se and the influence of characteristics that tend to occur more frequently with greater age but are important no matter when they occur.

This is not a unique problem. While it is still debated, and there is evidence on both sides, there has been a question as to whether obesity is an independent cardiovascular risk, or whether the elevated blood pressure, blood sugar, and cholesterol associated with obesity (or perhaps obesity — provoking diet) are the only risk factors. To give the best possible advice one needs to know the answer.

4. We are usually not wise enough in advance to know where to look for trouble. Therefore, in addition to looking at identified trouble areas, we need to set in place mechanisms to find the unexpected.

5. There is no insurmountable obstacle to including the elderly, in fairly sizable numbers, in clinical trials. We know this because patients in their 60s and 70s have regularly been included in evaluations of drugs in recent years (as a minisurvey of recent NDAs showed). Beyond the 70s it may become difficult as increasing problems can be expected to arrive from such mundane matters as reaching the clinic, assuring compliance with medications, obtaining informed consent, and so on. Note that I have given no age at which people become "elderly." In part that is because no one is likely to agree, and in part because the idea that people switch categories all at once is naive. Somewhere between 60 and 80 it happens to us all. NDAs should include a good representation of patients in this age range.

The solution that arose from these premises is somewhat complicated, with several components, reflecting an attempt to study those areas that we know are likely to cause problems in the elderly, study the basic properties of drugs better than we have in the past, and examine the rich data base of an NDA as well as possibly to discover new information.

We did not think it was enough simply to say: If the drug is to be used in the elderly, carry out clinical trials and a pharmacokinetic study in old people. It seemed almost inevitable that such studies would be carried out in a relatively healthy elderly population, with special care devoted to dose selection, and would show little except the usual response. These studies may be useful sometimes, but are not sufficient. Accepting them as sufficient would, I think, be deceiving ourselves.

We therefore proposed the following set of requirements, some related specifically to the elderly, others to obtaining general information that will be useful to all age groups including the elderly.

BETTER STUDY OF FACTORS KNOWN
TO ALTER PHARMACOKINETICS

It appears at this time that a substantial fraction of the drug problems in the elderly have to do with alterations in the pharmacokinetics of drugs. It is not well enough recognized that changes in creatinine clearance (CCr) are very common in the elderly and accurate clearances are hard to obtain, as they require 24-hour urine collections. There is a simple formula developed by Cockcroft and Gault:

$$\text{Male CCr} = \frac{\text{wt (kg)} \times (140 - \text{age})}{72 \times \text{Cr (mg/100 ml)}}$$

$$\text{Female CCr} = 0.9 \times \text{above}$$

For most purposes, the formula gives an estimate superior to any but the most meticulous measurements. Marc Reidenberg informed me of his recent study in hospitalized patients comparing the estimate using the above equation and actual CCr measurements. Whenever there was a meaningful difference between the estimate and the measurement, repeat of the measurement gave a value closer to the calculated value than to the previous measured value.

In addition to knowing CCr, we must know how the kinetics of the drug are affected by changes in renal function. Therefore, any drug excreted (parent drug or active metabolites) through renal mechanisms should have formal study of the effect of altered renal function or its pharmacokinetics. Labeling for such drugs should portray this relationship and include the Cockcroft and Gault equation above, or provide a nomogram equivalent. This is clearly possible, as it already is done for the aminoglycosides, a renally excreted class of drugs with a very narrow therapeutic ratio.

The proposal suggested routine study of the influence of protein binding on kinetics, but several comments cast doubt on the usefulness of this.

The proposal did not mention purely biopharmaceutic matters, but there is growing interest in such factors as pH dependence of dosage forms and effects of delayed gastric emptying. The elderly are more likely to be hypochlorhydric and to have delayed emptying.

The proposal did not consider relating kinetics to hepatic function such as might be assessed by an aminopyrine test, but Dr Greenblatt's paper suggests potential usefulness of such an effort (see Chapter 20). The problem, obviously, is that relatively few physicians utilize an aminopyrine test as part of their clinical dose-selection procedures, so that identifying a relationship might be of little practical value.

A SCREEN FOR UNKNOWN/UNSUSPECTED PHARMACOKINETIC EFFECTS

The proposal includes a "pharmacokinetic screen," a procedure involving obtaining a small number of blood samples during steady state dosing from many patients to look for unexpectedly high or low blood levels.

At present, pharmacokinetic studies are carried out principally in small numbers of normal males. Only if obvious problems develop are searches made in other populations, except that kinetics in patients with abnormal renal function are fairly commonly studied and certain specific drug interaction studies (eg, effects on digoxin or crystalline warfarin sodium [Coumadin]) are increasingly common.

If there is a suitable blood level assay, preferably one not too dependent on perfect handling of samples, blood levels obtained during clinical trials should be able to detect major deviations from what is expected. Once detected, the reasons for the deviation must be sought among the usual factors, such as:

• demographic characteristics (age, race, sex)

• effects of other disease (hepatic function, CHF)

• effects of other drugs (cimetidine, barbiturates)

• population differences in metabolism (isoniazid, procaine amide, encainide)

• unrecognized peculiar kinetics (nonlinearity)

The proposal suggested that several blood levels would be needed to define approximate peak and trough levels. One comment, from Dr Reidenberg, who was concerned that the suggestion was needlessly burdensome, suggested that trough levels alone would suffice, for several reasons:

• trough and peak are related

• the usual clinical correlations of drug effect are with trough levels

• peak will be hard to find and requires arbitrary choices

Obviously, it would be substantially easier to obtain trough levels only. Timing would be less critical and fewer samples needed. This bears further discussion.

Dr Reidenberg also suggested that the screen could be omitted if certain conditions obtained (eg, if a drug was eliminated wholly as the unmetabolized parent compound by the kidneys, the renal work-up might suffice). Or, if a drug had an easily measured, rapid response clearly related to dose (some antihypertensive agents) one might know well enough how to use it from the kinds of studies now carried out. These points too bear further discussion.

Let me emphasize that a "screen" is a hypothesis-generating device, not usually able to provide a definitive answer. If outliers are found, their characteristics (age, race, disease, other drugs, obesity, etc) need to be examined to seek an explanation and further studies in them could be needed. It would also be important to determine whether the observed drug responses in outliers (effects, adverse drug reactions) were different, as it is the clinical importance of a pharmacokinetic alteration that is our real concern.

STUDIES OF PHARMACOKINETIC INTERACTIONS

There are a few formal studies of drug-drug interaction that probably should be part of any drug evaluation (eg, effects on digoxin serum levels) and some studies are suggested by the way drugs will be used (eg, antianginal and anti-congestive heart failure [anti-CHF] drugs will be used together and should be studied together), but a screening mechanism seems useful here, again concentrating on pharmacokinetic interactions first. Proposed is a simple comparison of trough, steady-state blood levels before and after introduction of the new drug. Obviously, this can be done most readily where the institution is already capable of monitoring blood levels of a particular drug and setting up many new assays would be prohibitively costly. It is often, of course, the drugs whose levels are most critical (phenytoin, quinidine, digoxin, etc) that hospitals choose to measure, so that the screen would be targeted to agents of major interest.

SPECIAL AGE-RELATED REQUIREMENTS

As noted, the above requirements would greatly enhance knowledge of drugs pertinent to the elderly but are pertinent to all patients.

Several additional requirements are needed:

1. Drugs should be explicitly described with respect to how likely their use in the elderly is. This may be self-evident from the target population (CHF and angina, eg, obviously are common in older patients) but, if not, can be derived from sources such as Medicaid or the National Disease and Therapeutic Index.

2. Elderly patients should be included in clinical trials. They usually are, at present, but sometimes there are arbitrary age limits (eg, patients over 75) that seem of doubtful necessity. Caution, especially early, is understandable, but by Phase III older patients should be included.

The proposal does not call for routine specific clinical studies in the elderly, but suggests that the elderly be included in other trials as they appear. Clearly, however, for drugs very specifically targeted to the elderly or where differences in response by age might be expected (eg, sedatives), trials in the elderly could be carried out or, even better, response in old and young could be specifically compared. The paper by Dr Greenblatt (see Chapter 20) suggests that it would be appropriate to carry out pharmacokinetic studies of any high-clearance oxidized drug in the elderly.

3. Adverse effects and effectiveness should be analyzed by age. I am impressed that we do not sufficiently use the mass of data in an NDA to look for factors that affect response, factors such as age, race, dose (in mg/kg), other diseases, other drugs, obesity, or blood level. I recognize that cross-study pooling of data for such an analysis is risky, but there is no possibility of gaining these insights in any other way unless someone is smart enough

to suspect such a relationship. Certainly, suspected relationships should be pursued, but sifting the data for surprises is also of value.

It should be obvious that we are proposing no "cookbook," but rather an approach. Some commentators preferred an alternative suggested by Crooks, one now possibly being used in England. The alternative is to identify drugs likely to create problems in the elderly:

• Drugs intended for indications commonly found in the elderly

• Drugs with low therapeutic ratio and either: (a) renally excreted, (b) having a high liver extraction ratio, (c) acting on the CNS, or (d) having an effect likely to be modified by the impairment of homeostatic mechanisms commonly found in the elderly

For these, three studies would be needed:

• Single-dose pharmacokinetic studies in healthy older patients (70 years old)

• Pharmacodynamic studies in elderly patients with the disease to be treated

• Establishment of safety and effectiveness in the elderly using trial conditions suggested by the above results

The proposal has merit and may represent a reasonable minimum effort. Its problem, I think, is that it focuses on age alone. I do not believe, and, more important, the gerontologists who write about drugs and the elderly do not indicate, that the specific effect of age is the biggest problem. The biggest problem is the effect of age in causing a variety of diseases and system impairment and need for other drugs resulting in a wide range of interactions. The above studies, carried out in a fairly healthy older population will tell about the specific effects of age but will leave the elderly unguarded against problems that arise not from age itself but from age-related impairments of excretion, need for other therapy, and concomitant illness. I believe the broader approach proposed, refined by comments from within and outside the FDA, though perhaps more difficult to implement, has greater promise.

The next step, after reviewing all comments, and perhaps convincing groups to discuss specific issues, will be to propose guidelines, probably presented as a series of specific amendments to our General Guidelines. I hope anyone interested will comment as soon as possible so that the proposed guideline is the best possible document. The most effective comments are those that include specific alternatives.

Chapter 23

INVESTIGATIONAL
NEW DRUG TRIALS
IN GERIATRIC SUBJECTS

Frances O. Kelsey, MD, PhD

The rapidly increasing proportion of elderly persons in the population has emphasized the need for safe and effective drugs for geriatric patients. Recognizing that there may be age-related differences in reactions to drugs, it can be anticipated that an increasing number of investigational new drug studies involving older subjects will be undertaken as sponsors seek to provide information pertaining to the use of their products in this age group. Such studies raise certain scientific and ethical problems that must be faced by the sponsor, the clinical investigator, and the FDA.

The Division of Scientific Investigations has encountered a number of such problems in its review of studies at over 30 geriatric nursing homes conducted by some 17 clinical investigators or investigational teams. In addition, we have reviewed a few outpatient studies involving geriatric patients. I will describe the FDA's investigational program in the drug area and inspectional findings as they apply to elderly subjects in this chapter.

Fundamental measures for the protection of human subjects of clinical studies include well qualified investigators with adequate facilities and well designed and properly executed clinical studies preceded by adequate preclinical studies. Additional important safeguards are afforded by truly informed patient consent and by initial and continuing review of the study by an institutional review board (IRB). The FDA requires that before starting investigational drug studies clinical investigators must sign a commitment to the sponsor, Forms FD 1572 or FD 1573, with regard to the proper conduct of the trial, including the obtaining of patient consent and institutional review board approval. The sponsor of the drug study (usually the manufacturer) in turn makes commitments to the FDA (as set forth in Form FD 1571) to develop well designed protocols to evaluate safety and efficacy, to select appropriate clinical investigators, to inform them of their responsibilities under the regulations, and to monitor the conduct of studies to assure compliance with the regulations. The FDA has an obligation to ensure that protocols adequately protect the safety of subjects; that clinical investigators are qualified in the respective field of study; and that all other regulatory requirements are met by sponsors, investigators, and institutional review boards.

Inspections of the work of clinical investigators in order to determine their compliance with regulations were started in the drug area, albeit in a limited way, in 1962. A program of inspections of preclinical laboratories was begun in 1971 and institutional review board inspections were started in 1974. Deficiencies noted in these early inspections were largely responsible for the development in 1977 of an agency-wide Bioresearch Monitoring Program, under which inspections are made of clinical investigators, institutional review boards, and laboratories conducting nonclinical (animal) studies. The Division of Scientific Investigations is responsible for the Bioresearch Monitoring Program in the drug area.

Under this program, the Clinical Investigations Branch of the division directs three types of inspections of clinical investigators. The first of these is the routine surveillance inspection. Approximately 200 clinical investigators are visited each year under this program, selection being on the basis of a stratified sampling system. Of highest priority for inspection are studies deemed important to the acceptance of a new drug application undergoing agency review. Other categories are studies submitted in support of new claims for marketed drugs, studies done under mature INDs, efficacy studies done to upgrade claims for drugs approved between 1938 and 1962 on the basis of safety only, studies submitted in support of over-the-counter drugs, and finally studies done under noncommercial INDs.

Routine investigations are conducted by FDA field investigators and consist of two basic parts. The first part is the evaluation of the physician's conduct of the study, including the degree of delegation of authority, how and where data were recorded; and how the drug substance was accounted for. A determination is also made of whether and to what degree the sponsor monitored the study. The second part of the routine investigation is the audit of data. Here the FDA investigator compares the data submitted to the agency with the data in the records on site.

A second type of clinical investigation inspection is the so-called "for cause" inspection. In most "for cause" inspections, a headquarters scientist accompanies the field investigator. Such an inspection may be triggered by a number of factors and does not necessarily indicate any suspicion of wrongdoing. Inspections may be done of investigators doing a large volume of work outside their field of specialty or because the investigator has done work that merits in-depth examination due to its singular importance. Approximately 5% of routine inspections reveal problems sufficiently serious to prompt an in-depth inspection. "For cause" inspections are also triggered by complaints received from sponsors, from hospital or clinic personnel, or from subjects or relatives of subjects. A number of such complaints have been directed towards studies involving geriatric patients.

The third type of data audit undertaken by the division is that of a bioavailability study. In this program, the analytical facility is audited as well as the clinical facility, and for this reason a chemist knowledgeable of the analytical procedure participates in the inspection. Some 20 such inspections are conducted annually. To date, subjects in these studies have been young male volunteers. This may change if bioavailability studies serve as a basis of approval for geriatric drug claims.

The number of geriatric studies that we have audited to date is too small to permit any sweeping conclusions. However, some observations can be offered at this time, particularly with regard to patient consent; inadequate, inaccurate, and unavailable records; and absence of or improper institutional board review.

Informed consent has been a requirement of investigational drug studies since the 1962 Kefauver-Harris Amendment of the Food, Drug and Cosmetic Act. A recent (1981) revision of the regulations gives clear and precise directions as to the required elements of patient consent and requires that all consent for investigational new drug use be obtained in writing. Exemption from the requirement of informed consent is permissible only if the following four conditions obtain: the subject's condition is life threatening, the subject is incapable of giving consent, there is no time to obtain consent from the subject's legal representative, and there is no other available nonexperimental therapy that provides equal or greater likelihood of saving the life of the subject.

Inadequacy in the informed consent process is the most common deficiency in clinical investigator inspections, being noted in roughly 50% of routine inspections. It should be emphasized that in these cases only rarely was consent not obtained. In most instances, the deficiency was omission of one or more of the required essential elements of consent and, on occasion, the inclusion of exculpatory language, which is specifically prohibited by the regulations. Some serious deficiencies have been found, however, in the consent procedures in geriatric studies during both routine and "for cause" inspections. Consent forms have been signed by subjects, sometimes in the form of an "X," although the subject's hospital record clearly indicated he or she did not have the mental capacity to give informed consent. In other cases, approval for the subject to enter a study was given by an individual other than the legally authorized representative. Often, consent forms could not be located in patient records and thus it could not be established that consent had been obtained.

An important aspect of the consent process is the understanding that a subject is free to withdraw from a trial without prejudice. Inspections have however uncovered instances in which, even after the geriatric subject (or legal representative) refused a dose or requested withdrawal from the study, the investigational drug continued to be given, disguised in food. Justification given was that this was a standard procedure in nursing homes. While such a procedure may or may not be justified for a marketed drug, it is quite inappropriate for an investigational drug. It is recognized that subjects in drug studies from time to time refuse to take a dose. All missed doses must be recorded in the case report forms, so that the sponsor and FDA medical officers and statisticians can take such occurrences into account. However, surreptitious administration of an investigational drug is improper and the right of a subject to withdraw from a study must remain intact.

Because of the importance of obtaining consent the principal investigator should undertake this task himself or herself rather than delegate it to a junior member of the research team. However, if the authority for obtaining informed consent is delegated, the investigator must determine that the person obtaining the consent is fully conversant with the nature of the clinical trial and the rights of the subject and must verify in some appropriate way that the delegated activities have been discharged in a responsible fashion. We believe that total delegation is improper, and that the responsible physician must have some meaningful contact with each subject.

In most of the audited geriatric studies, the principal investigator was not the primary care physician of the subjects in the clinical trial. This was true for both nursing home studies and outpatient studies when subjects were obtained through referral or other means such as by advertisement. In some nursing home studies, the investigator had no connection with the institution other than through the performance of the trial or trials. Nursing home management, the subject's family, or the subject's primary physician were not always fully cognizant of the nature of the trial. Because the investigator was not responsible for primary care, he or she had little or no control over the administration of concomitant medications and patients' charts usually contained scanty if any reference to the ongoing trial. Psychometric or other tests were administered by study nurses who likewise were independent of the institution and had no day-to-day contact with subjects.

Current FDA regulations require that all investigational drug studies, whether conducted in an institution or in a private office, be reviewed and approved and be subject to continuing review by an institutional review board (IRB). In virtually all geriatric studies reviewed, if there was any in-house review of the protocol, it was likely to have been by a utilization review committee rather than an institutional review board as defined in the regulations. Although the IRB requirements do not specifically address drug trials in the aged, the regulations do require that "if an IRB regularly reviews research that involves a vulnerable category of subjects, including but not limited to subjects covered by other parts of this chapter, the IRB should include one or more individuals who are primarily concerned with the welfare of these subjects."

Factors that might make geriatric subjects vulnerable would include the mental status of the subjects, the absence of family support, the overdependence on institutional care (which might make it difficult for them to refuse study participation), the presence of other illness, and the possible language barriers to understanding the informed consent document.

At the present time, there is no requirement that the sponsor identify to the agency the institutional review board (IRB) that will review a particular drug protocol. Proposed revision of the investigational new drug regulations will require the sponsor to furnish this information, which will enable the agency to develop a more efficient system of identifying IRBs and scheduling inspections. It should also permit the agency to better direct educational efforts towards the less experienced IRBs.

While sponsors may not always direct specific attention to the elderly, older patients are often included in drug studies. Many protocols do, however, specify an upper age limit for subjects, commonly 60 or 65 years. But when such studies are audited, it is not unusual to find that, although the case report forms indicate all patients fell in the appropriate range, hospital or clinic records may show some well outside of the range. Inclusion of such patients is usually defended on the basis that they met the requirements in all other respects and that age was not necessarily a contraindication to a given drug. However, such liberties of interpretation mean that important data with regard to effect of a drug in the geriatric age group may be lost. Subjects are thus put at risk without the data being presented in the manner that would provide accurate information to the sponsor and to the agency. In the absence of specific contraindications, removal of upper age limits for studies of drugs that if approved for marketing will be used in elderly subjects would obviate this duplicity and provide needed information.

In conclusion, our inspections point to deficiencies in investigational drug studies as currently conducted in the elderly. It is apparent that, in general, nursing homes do not provide the environment necessary to conduct adequate and well controlled and much-needed clinical trials. However, exceptions do exist, particularly in well supported, long-term care institutions serving a stable population and with a staff of well trained physicians and nurses. The development of the teaching nursing home concept may provide further opportunities. Confounding factors to drug studies in the elderly include the frequency of coexisting disease conditions requiring concomitant therapy, the difficulty in diagnosing certain specific disease entities, and, often, the reluctance of the aged to enter or to continue in such studies. Although many of these difficulties can be circumvented through simpler approaches, such as bioavailability studies, there will remain the need for actual clinical trials of drugs designed to treat conditions peculiar to the elderly. The demographic changes of our population necessitate the development of more sophisticated research centers and research protocols designed to study the particular problems unique to the geriatric population.

PART 9

HEALTH PROMOTION FOR THE ELDERLY

Chapter 24

PIONEERING IN HEALTH PROMOTION: REACHING THE ELDERLY

J. Michael McGinnis, MD

Think for a moment of this contrast: first, the patient who has just been told that his disease is incurable, terminal, and hopeless; then, the patient who is told he has a minor, passing problem that will improve if a few simple steps are taken. It takes no special prescience to predict a better outcome for the second patient — regardless of the disease. All too often in our society, aging has been treated as a terminal condition, a hopeless disease, a state without cure. Indeed, aging is a life process frequently perceived not only negatively but fearfully as early as the third decade of life. No other human condition, no other phase of life, is so misunderstood. It's time for a hard look at the evidence on aging. With even passing scrutiny, we can see that scars we may take as signs of aging are, in fact, more directly the sequelae of disease than inevitable consequences of the aging process.

Our attitudes toward aging are so negative, so pervasive, that they surround and permeate our actions. The mere mention of health promotion for the elderly is more likely to bring tolerant smiles than hearty enthusiasm.

We need to weed out attitudes that are defeating. In a sense our focus on the inevitable declines that occur with age is a manifestation of lack of appreciation of the complexity and adaptability of a human being. It is truly a case of seeing the glass as half empty instead of half full. Yet, even the half that remains is in most cases more than sufficient for full enjoyment of our daily lives. There can be no doubt that an enormous opportunity exists to improve the quality of life for many if we can break out of old patterns and biases. But these are tenacious biases and they permeate the attitudes of even our elderly. Studies have shown that older people expect physical discomfort as they age. People say, "I feel very young for my age." Gloria Steinem once made a stir when she responded to a remark that she didn't look 40, by saying "This is what 40 looks like." We need a new appreciation of what 40, 50, 60, 70, and even 80 "look like." Individuals are sensing that the stereotypes are wrong and scientists are proving it. There is probably no group so ready for a new attitude about life, no group so in need of health information and encouragement, no group so in need of shedding therapeutic fatalism, as those among us who are the older Americans.

Think for a moment how different our approaches and attitudes would be if we treated all 65-year-olds as if they were 25. We would naturally encourage them to do all kinds of things to protect and promote their health. There would be no slowing down allowed — certainly not for 25-year-olds. If illness or injury occurred, optimism and the most active interventions would be encouraged. These young patients would be encouraged to take an interest in their own medical care, to ask questions, and to know and understand the effects of the medications deployed. Contrast that to the way such problems would be treated in 70-year-olds.

Hopefully, we are now on the way to finding out that health can be maintained until a period shortly before death. Scientists at Harvard have introduced a new term, "active life expectancy." This phrase is exciting as it moves from a mere calculation of life expectancy, of the biological limits of life, estimated by a few brave researchers to be about 110 to 120 years, to a more fundamental appreciation of the issue of quality of life. It is the period of disability and decline at the end of life that is the time feared by all mankind, not the extension of the productive and healthy middle years. "Active life expectancy" takes into account dimensions of health and morbidity other than death — a compelling concept for policymakers, researchers, and health care professionals.

Today, one in nine Americans is over 65, and in 35 years we expect one in five to be in that age group. Today, this group numbers 26 million and will almost triple in size to 77 million by 2035. Today nearly 80% of Americans 65 or older have at least one chronic health problem. But the fact is that most report little or no difficulty in living normal lives. The most common problems are arthritis, hypertension, hearing loss, visual loss, and heart problems — conditions with the potential, in many cases, to respond to exercise, nutrition, and good early care.

In 1983 our total U.S. health care costs were projected at more than $360 billion. More than 1 out of 10 dollars spent today goes to health expenditures. Older Americans accounted for 30% of the health care spending in the United States, 40% of acute hospital billings, and 90% of the cost of nursing home care. Yet many of the chronic diseases inflicting these burdens may be prevented or diminished. Even in devastating illnesses such as Alzheimer's disease there is growing evidence that the decline can be slowed. Better diagnostic techniques have shown that some patients remain on a plateau rather than plunging further into mental confusion. To date we do not know why, but if this mystery yields to research, and there is every sign that it eventually will, the social and economic gains will be dramatic.

The Massachusetts study offers impressive expectations for active lives for older people. It suggests that people entering the age group 65 to 69 have 10 active years ahead, those entering the 80 to 84 group have nearly 5 years, and about 3 years remain for those 85 and older. We have a growing indication that our older years can be active and productive years. And this is the case for an expanding segment of our society.

Interviews under the direction of my staff have shown that the elderly are very eager to learn and to make changes where necessary in their daily patterns to enhance their health. Their interest is avid. Evidence is accumulating to reinforce this observation. A study of 20,000 consumers in four ambulatory care facilities showed that they were just as prepared to follow health care advice as a younger group. But our initiative with these people is often quelled by our entrenched expectations of decline.

I think one cannot overemphasize the importance of factoring the needs of older Americans into our national goals and aspirations.

In 1979 the Surgeon General issued a report entitled *Healthy People*. Among the objectives for the older population was the intent to reduce the average annual number of days of restricted activity among the elderly by 20% to fewer than 30 days per year. Implicit is the goal of delaying the onset of illness and doing all possible to maintain the functioning of the already ill. Our broader hope is to improve the quality of life for older Americans.

We are taking this challenge seriously and making good progress. A major health promotion initiation under the direction of my staff has identified some key areas for special activity designed to achieve these goals and improve life for the elderly: injury prevention, physical fitness, nutrition, smoking, alcohol and drug education, and preventive health services.

No one suggests that we will eliminate disease in old age. But just as we learned to understand the natural history of diseases such as tuberculosis and typhoid, and to purify water and improve sanitation, we need to learn now about the effects on health outcomes of lifelong habits and exposures. We need, and are rapidly accumulating, baseline information about the physiology of the older person. A better understanding of the timetable needed for effective interventions, in some cases years before clinical onset, may be needed in some diseases.

So, although we do not anticipate eliminating disease or disability, we have some tantalizing suggestions about how to reduce them. Clearly, any such effort must be directed to the problems of appropriate use of medications for and by the elderly. These issues touch on problems of drug interaction, the precise use of medications in a population with accumulated diseases and disabilities, and establishing the risks or benefits of food and water additives, as well as micronutrients such as vitamins and minerals. We need to know more about the way the elderly self-prescribe and how to encourage intelligent compliance. Here the issue of health promotion must be viewed as a dual challenge to the health provider and lay participant alike. All too often the elderly confer such blind trust upon their physicians that they literally do not know the medications they are consuming. In an era of multiple specialists treating the same patient, the responsibility for coordinating medical care often falls between the cracks, leaving a confused consumer the task of questioning practices he or she has come to regard as sacred. A new enlightened attitude and partnership must be encouraged between patient, physician, and pharmacist.

But there are other problems. For example, alcohol use may pose special problems for the elderly. No good estimates exist of how many older people have significant problems with drinking, but some claim the figure may be as high as 10%. If a person has diabetes, heart disease, liver disease, or central nervous system impairment, he or she may suffer great harm with even a relatively modest amount of alcohol. Metabolic processes change with age, including those that metabolize the ethanol molecule. The need for "quality calories" in the older years is well recognized, and one encouraging sign is that some older people cite "cutting down on alcohol" as a means of weight control. But the recognition that alcohol may crowd out good food is not nearly as widespread as we would like. There is additional reason for concern as interactions with alcohol and medications commonly taken by the elderly are particularly dangerous. The average older person takes up to 13 medications a year, and not only are some of these medications dangerous mixtures but, if they are compounded by the use of alcohol, the results can be fatal.

Nutrition is a complex subject. We need to identify the special dietary needs of the elderly and how they vary with exercise and other substances ingested. Food has emotional meaning as well as dietary and social implications. Contrast the meal eaten with good friends in a pleasant room with a lonely snack.

Not all problems have to do with personal management of health care or with lifestyle issues. Some have to do with prompt application and dissemination of promising new scientific findings. Research now suggests that it is possible to push back the age-of-onset of osteoporosis — to retard the disease that thins and weakens the bones of older persons, particularly older women. We can delay or avoid many of the 200,000 annual cases of costly and painful hip fractures that so often result from this disease. Researchers at the National Institute on Aging are examining combinations of vitamins, increased calcium intake, and intensified and continued exercise, as well as judicious use of estrogens, as factors that may be of assistance. In the meantime, there is much to be gained from encouraging women in their 30s and 40s to expand their calcium intake and to exercise.

But to encourage people to exercise we need to break through a certain fatalism. A 1975 survey showed that only 36% of adults aged 65 and over took regular walks — this in spite of the fact that there are many mild forms of exercise such as walking or swimming that can be safely undertaken, even when one is in fragile health. Other reports suggest that exercise can also be beneficial to the bedridden or chairbound. Health scientists have understood and acted on the research that showed the risks of bedrest. Now we get people up as soon as possible, even after major surgery. We need to go further, both literally and figuratively. Dr Robert Butler, Director of the National Institute on Aging, captured the spirit succinctly when he said: "If exercise could be packed into a pill, it would be the single most widely prescribed and beneficial medicine in the nation." Movement is life. Old adages such as "use it or lose it" are turning out to be far more than folk wisdom.

But there are prominent attitudinal barriers and misinformation. The survey of older people we are now undertaking indicates that one of the disincentives to their participation is fear of increasing their heart or respiratory rate — the very effect needed for conditioning. We must seek out and overcome these biases.

Another promising area for gain is in the prevention of accidental injuries. The death rate for injuries is higher for people 75 and older than for any other group. They are harmed by falls, fires, burns, suffocation, poisoning by gases and vapors, and motor vehicle accidents. Accidents in 1977 accounted for almost 43 million days of bed disability. We need more research to learn how to teach older people to alter their driving patterns, to adjust to slower reaction times and diminished visual acuity.

Going back to our example of 65-year-olds masquerading as 25-year-olds, consider our advice on smoking. In spite of the fact that smoking poses a very serious threat, not only from the substantial, and sometimes irreversible, pathophysiologic damage it inflicts, but as the dominant source of fatal fires, often we are reluctant to push for smoking cessation by older adults. In the spirit of asking older adults to do as much as possible to improve and maintain their health, this must be changed.

I know what I hope for as I grow older. I wish, as all of us do, to have the opportunity to continue to participate, to continue to develop and learn, and to continue to offer what expertise I have. I want my health to be good, and I want the best information as fast as possible so that I can exercise my own judgment about protecting my life. I want to live with my family and continue to care for the people I love.

After I reach age 65, I certainly do not want to spend the last 17 years of my life in passive resignation and uneasy acceptance of unnecessary decline. I wish for a full and active lifestyle and I wish these benefits for all other Americans as well. I want to urge embarking on a new era of concern for the elderly, with deliberate attention to the pressing research needs associated with aging and a commitment to aggressive and clear communication of health information. In the Public Health Service we have a unique blend of the finest research and the ability to reach all Americans. We have a proud history of fighting disease and are making a commendable record in promoting health. As a nation, we have an outstanding record in developing and testing new drugs. Dissemination of information must be linked to research. Let us make clear our conviction that true health is more than an absence of disease, it is a total state of activity and awareness. As health professionals, let us all join to work on behalf of the elderly and move quickly to shed old attitudes and practices. Let us redouble our effort to add life to those extra years we're promoting for all Americans of all ages.

PART 10

INDUSTRY INVOLVEMENT IN GERIATRIC DRUG USE

Chapter 25

AN OVERVIEW
OF INDUSTRY ACTIVITIES
AND DRUG USE IN THE ELDERLY

Hugh H. Tilson, MD, PhD

When we discuss directions for "the industry" we're referring to a very heterogeneous group of companies. Some companies are heavily research-based; some are not heavily research-based. Some are involved in one drug or one small segment of the market; some are involved in many. Some are deeply involved in basic science; some are simply involved in drug development. All are concerned with regulatory matters, not wishing to be held inappropriately accountable for things they cannot control and, on the other hand, still wishing to be accountable and responsible. All have commercial and proprietary concerns: "We can't talk too much about too many things too soon because things may not pan out; or there are patent concerns; or there are company images involved." Those are all legitimate concerns for an epidemiologist looking at geriatric issues in the industry, as I have been for the last 3 months. And they apply equally in the area of aging. There are also legal concerns. Others speaking to the subject have suggested there probably isn't much of a problem with lawsuits in geriatric drug use. I don't know any area in health care where there is not a major problem with lawsuits in 1984.

What I've tried to do is put together a few illustrations about industry activities with regard to aging that are relatively in the public arena, although many companies have been extraordinarily generous in sharing them with me.

What does one do when there aren't any answers to the questions that one needs to ask? As an epidemiologist I did the only thing I could do, and that is I asked. I resorted to a survey because I tried to find the answers in the literature, or in other surveys, or by simply putting together the pieces of information that I had or that are in the heads of the other people around the tables where I routinely eat lunch. But nobody seemed to know. Thus, this survey was conceived to begin to fill a void in our information about the level and scale of current industry contribution to addressing the problems of aging. It's not a very good survey.

Epidemiologists need always to go through the biases in their surveys. In this survey each of the representatives of the drug companies who chose to come to this workshop was asked to complete a mailed questionnaire. Now, of course, that is a very biased sample. They were likely to be companies having some specific activity involving drugs and the elderly or thinking about some. Given that as a bias, of the 20 companies contacted, 17 responded. Of course, as with many such surveys, particularly those done by an epidemiologist, the survey asked the wrong questions. For example, it asked "Has your company created a 'program' for pharmaceutical issues for the elderly?" trying to get a handle on what the industry is doing. Of the 17 companies that responded to the question "Do you have a program on aging?" about half said yes and half said no. That question was utterly unrelated to the rest of the information in the questionnaire; it was the wrong question. Epidemiologists tend to think in terms of program. But people in the industry don't always do this. It was the wrong question because of the 17 replies, only 2 failed to give information that sounded like "a program" in working on drugs for the elderly. The important news from this survey is: If the "generic exhortation" is applied point by point to the drug industry it can be seen that substantively on each count we are "on the right track."

Specifically, for example, in the area of development of necessary drugs, marketing, quality assurance, and maintenance of that quality over time, drug companies are exceedingly aware of the issues here and address them all the time. Pharmaceutical products for the elderly are, first and foremost, pharmaceuticals. They require and receive the same careful attention as all others. When drugs are developed for use in the older population, elders are, in fact, included in drug testing today. In all of the companies contacted (except two, which don't yet market drugs particularly involved in chronic disease control that would be taken by elders), when elders were predicted to be among major users, drugs were tested in those elders. I'm not suggesting that the companies report that they think they did everything they could have. I'm not even suggesting that they think they did everything in every case they should have. Those are the wrong things to assume always. We will always leave undone some things that we need to have done. But rather, the question is one of the good faith and cost/effectiveness of what they do. At the least, I'm very pleased to report that of the companies I contacted virtually all are reassessing, reevaluating on the bases of new and emergent interest in drugs and the elderly, whether in fact they have already done enough with the drugs that they have marketed and are continuing to do enough with the drugs that they are now testing. Those are questions for which the answers are yet to come in.

Regarding the question of a "program," in one company, the person contacted said no to Question 1 initially and reported later that after three hours he found the person who was running the program and the answer should have been yes. That tells you something about the complexity of describing the length and breadth of industry involvement in specific issues with the elderly and of understanding programming in general in a large and complex industry.

Regarding new drugs under development, there is an extraordinary story, one that can't be told entirely, certainly not in the space of an article, nor is it appropriate in the public forum to do some of the telling that could be done. The industry has a heavy investment — some 17 companies over $20 million and four over $100 million a year — in basic science and drug development. There is an extraordinary dollar investment in the bringing of new and newly needed drugs into a marketplace where the people we've been talking about, about whom we all care, the elderly, can benefit from them. There is a fine line between basic research and drug development. Many companies report extraordinary programs in basic sciences, trying to understand the mechanisms of disease and of the biology of the elderly so that they can develop new drugs in that area. They all report that which you already know: the Ponce de Leon Syndrome is not going to obtain, nor is there going to be a silver bullet, nor do most of the diseases and problems of the elderly have single etiologies. We are in a new world with aging in which for the most part we're developing drugs against chronic disease; the industry is keenly aware of the multifactorial problems in trying basic etiologic research in getting at the treatments for those diseases. Nevertheless, even in this modest survey, there were major discovery and development programs in arthritis control, in lipid-lowering agents, in antithrombotics, and in lifestyle questions — not just the antidepressants and the anxiolytics, but in sexual and social function, for example, of the elderly. Those avenues of research are being aggressively pursued in drug companies today. Perhaps the most exciting for those of us who can't remember names and addresses even in our mid-40s is in the area of cognition and memory, where over half of the respondents said that they had "something doing" in the area. Now, obviously, there is a long way to go before we have drugs that can actually address these problems, although some companies have been much more successful than others in bringing these drugs to clinical trial. Suffice it to say for the purposes of this inventory that the hope is great, and justified, for several major cognition- and memory-enhancing drugs to help us in a major way with the problems of senility and early institutionalization by the year 2000. The probability is very high for a major breakthrough.

On the delivery system side, there's much to be said concerning pharmaceutical industry activities and the aging. Delivery of services, after all, is critical. Just because we have needed cures doesn't mean that people can get to them. Just because people can get to them doesn't mean that they will understand, and just because they understand doesn't mean that they will comply, use, and be benefited. From the industry's reports, it is being very responsible in taking a look at the delivery system, trying to be part of the solutions to problems rather than causing them. As the health care delivery system itself evolves to introduce cost-containing activities (health maintenance organizations, for example), new drug distribution patterns have emerged with new wholesaling and retailing features. The pharmaceutical industry has been responding, trying to be sure that, whatever pattern is at work out there, the drug industry will be able to get pharmacuticals into the hands of those people who need the drugs.

Of course, on the microdelivery system level, trying to find creative packaging and ways of helping elders, the chronically ill, and disabled to gain better individual access to drugs is part of the challenge. Cost containment is an interesting dimension. Ask drug companies what they're doing to be part of the cost-containment aspect of our nation's escalating health care cost problem and they will report three things. We're manufacturing drugs, which will help people from becoming chronically ill and disabled and, therefore, institutionalized and part of the major cost component. We are trying to get those drugs out to people in the most cost-effective way we can. We are the sector of the industry that is more competitive and therefore, by competition and the attendant market mechanisms, we try to keep prices down. Now, there are aspects of that that would be interesting to debate. Suffice it to say that the proportion that pharmaceuticals play in the total cost of health care in our country has gone progressively down as the other segments of the industry have gone up to the point where now pharmaceuticals constitute 6.9% of the health care per person cost rather than 9.9% as they did 10 years ago. Concerning the problem of polypharmacy, creative packaging is needed, and the industry is exploring such approaches. Oral contraceptives, as far as I know, are not necessarily appropriate for the elderly in general terms, but the usefulness of creative packaging in this sphere (ie, daily dose wheels) can readily be seen for the chronic drug taker. The industry does know how to do that and is doing so. One clever package I found during the survey was a dose pack marked: "After breakfast, one; after supper, two"; and then the same for each day — third day, fourth day, and so on so that the person can be helped to figure out what to do with the complicated medication. Pill calendars and prescription-sized packages and blister packs are very useful ways for a person who has a very complicated pharmaceutical pattern to arrange his or her pill schedule, although I have yet to find one that will accommodate 11 medications at any one time during any one day. And, of course, you know that not all caps are childproof or foolproof. However, the industry has come up with some that even I can open, including one example sent with the survey in which the cap had "wings" to facilitate gripping.

A simple example shows what can be done in color change. One company provided the example of a yellow pill that was also developed at half the dose of the white one because it was found that the primary users of this particular medication had trouble breaking the scored white tablet, which you and I would not have a problem with, and so a smaller dose form in a different color was needed. And, when there was a problem in some patients with bioavailability, that same company went ahead and developed yet another more bioavailable compound, specifically for the aging and chronic heart disease population. The promotional materials for this product set a rather good example — showing *happy* chronic users, to show that at least old people can laugh even though they are chronically ill.

There is an enormous story to be told about the industry in education and collaboration. The educational efforts are quite remarkable. Actual examples were provided of materials directed at the problem of aging from about a dozen companies. Specific documents are produced by companies for each specific educational audience. Which audience? Well, it depends. The problem with drugs and the aging is that there are so many actors involved and so many of us making so many mistakes. Physicians, for example, face the barrage of information from "detailing" and "undetailing." The enormously clever approaches of many of our pharmaceutical houses have certainly succeeded in catching the doctors' attention. In the present survey, extraordinary resourcefulness was apparent in doing exactly that — packaging messages in a way that doctors, nurses, pharmacists, health workers, workers with the aging, and the public at large can understand. Universities and community health educators can learn much from the industry in this regard. Obviously, educating physicians about aging and not just drugs represents part of the agenda. One remarkable product comes from the Upjohn Company called the Psychopathology of Aging in their "current concepts" series. But I could have chosen examples from a number of companies; that one just happened to be the first on my bookshelf at the time. Another example of industry education of physicians is a reprinting of the *Family Practice Annual,* again issued by a grant from a pharmaceutical house; the last article in the 1981 edition was "Dementing Disorders of the Elderly"; and the last one in the 1982 edition was "Abuse of the Elderly," which included a section on pharmaceutical abuse and defacto imprisonment from over-drugging. General information for physicians and patients about various chronic diseases are the stock-in-trade of drug companies, but so is the presentation of scientific articles of high scholarship in areas that concern us all, published in the professional literature jointly with our university colleagues, with whom we in industry regularly collaborate and to whom we provide considerable amounts of money to help in the drug development enterprise. And seminars are sponsored for geriatric medicine as part of the continuing medical education programs of more than one pharmaceutical house. Journals, themselves, are another example of industry sponsorship, not just through advertising; for example, one major psychopharmacology journal happens to be edited by a person from a pharmaceutical house. And education for the population at large is widely undertaken by the industry on various aspects that are of interest to the aging. Regarding nutrition, and particularly the problem of accidents, for example, a set of abstracts has been generated by one company for public use. Education of patients is another major area where drug companies have done an extraordinary bit of work. For example, one major company (Roche) has generated a slide show that was put together for you and me or anybody who wants to reach the public. The slides are available, along with a script, and a document about how to present it. "What if the patient sees several doctors who prescribe medications?" Well, then, the guide says, answer about how to be an effective user of pharmaceuticals. And to strengthen the delivery system, another example from another drug company (Parke-Davis) is a program called "Elder Care" helping pharmacies to do education in the pharmacy. This particular company produces the slide show personalized for other organizations, not their own presentation — for example, it provides the Pharmacists' Association a "personalized" slide set to educate its own people about how to educate the patient. And from the industry itself, there are numerous collaborative efforts, for example in the Pharmaceutical Manufacturers Association or several other associational groups such as the National Pharmaceutical Council (NPC). Many drug companies participate cooperatively to develop and distribute information generally available to health care providers, consumers, and the public at large.

Regarding evaluation activity, our modest effort at taking stock prescribed here is fledgling, but we have to start somewhere. Nevertheless, we have punctuated our process and we now have made a beginning at getting a handle on just where the industry is and where it is going. I assume — no, I know — that this ongoing evaluation effort will continue.

But within the industry there is another major evaluation effort to which I want to call your attention. It is the vigor with which surveillance of adverse drug experiences in the elderly is being pursued by individual companies. Let me remind you, just to put it into perspective, that eight out of ten reports that come into the Food and Drug Administration for adverse drug experience monitoring are received, analyzed, investigated, processed, and reported by drug companies. It's as simple as that. I'm not suggesting we always do the very best job; I'm not suggesting that we're perfect. I am suggesting that we work hard and are committed to being part of the answers to proper monitoring for adverse drug experiences in the elderly. And, of course, one of the reasons for this chapter is the second part of that evaluation and accountability — namely, the emerging body of epidemiology within the industry. The assembly of programs in drug epidemiology now includes five companies in the industry of which I'm aware. These programs are looking not, incidentally, at an instant "fix" to the problems of adverse drug effects and not at applying some monolithic system of postmarketing surveillance that doesn't exist, nor at a single response to a major complicated scientific question, but rather at a complex, scientifically balanced approach to complex, scientific questions applying the right epidemiologic method to monitoring issues of prescription drug safety in the broader geriatric community. Of course, there are other aspects of pharmacoepidemiology emerging within the industry as well that I found out more about from my survey. The application of cost-benefit analysis techniques may help the industry to come up with a better shot at finding a way to make the drugs we know are needed, cost-effective, so that they can in fact come to the marketplace. On the subject of assessments of lifestyle and the implications and impact of our pharmaceuticals on the elderly, I found two excellent examples. And pharmacoepidemiologic programs are providing support of other aspects of service looking at drug use, drug distribution, and drug mishaps . . . all important geriatric drug issues.

We really can and must persevere in this commitment. After this survey we now know that there already is such commitment in the pharmaceutical industry and the industry doesn't need this exhortation from me to do what we already do. One hears, "We need to do it even better and to target the efforts at the highest priority." I can report that one of those highest priorities in the industry is drugs for the elderly, and that is exciting. Let me therefore summarize with three perspectives: In the area of research and development, it's clear that we will have new and needed drugs developed by the industry for the elderly; in the area of education, it's clear that we've already learned a lot from our own cleverness, particularly from the marketing side of companies, that can be applied to the general public; and, from those epidemiologists among us, I hope the industry is learning that there is reason to use the public health approach within pharmaceuticals particularly regarding drugs and the aging. But, again, this is an exhortation that's unneeded. The public health approach says we apply the principles of public health, namely the focus on outcomes, on populations, on accountability, and on prevention. And I guess one of the most startling parts of my survey is that I found that the words of our Surgeon General, Dr Koop, are prophetic in that they apply to the *actions* of industry in this area — namely that, in matters pertaining to the public health, cooperation and collaboration are the name of the game.

Chapter 26

DEVELOPMENT OF DRUGS FOR USE BY THE ELDERLY

William B. Abrams, MD

It is now well recognized that the elderly, defined as individuals over 65 years of age, are growing in numbers and as a proportion of the total population. It is also recognized that this group disproportionately uses medicines. At the present time, for example, the elderly represent about 11% of the population and are estimated to consume 20% to 25% of all medications.[1] Based on recent data from the U.S. Census Bureau, it is predicted that by 2030 the elderly will increase to about 21% of the U.S. population and consume more than 40% of all drugs. Equally important, the percentage growth of the "old elderly," those 75 or older, is even greater.[2] The high prevalence of disabilities in the very old increases the chances for therapeutic misadventures. Indeed, it is widely perceived that adverse drug reactions and drug interactions are more common in the elderly than in younger patients. A recent report of the Royal College of Physicians on adverse drug reactions in the elderly[3] identifies practices by treating physicians as central to this problem. On the other hand, a review by Klein et al[4] suggests the *incidence* of adverse drug reactions may not be greater in elderly patients but the *opportunity* certainly is.

Part of the problem resides in changes, mostly reductions, in many physiologic functions associated with the aging process. The principal changes are listed in Table 26.1. These changes have implications for drug disposition, and characteristic alterations in drug disposition have been described in elderly subjects (Table 26.2). In both tables the item of principal concern is the large variation that may be exhibited by this population. As noted above, the elderly are more likely to have multiple disorders and to take several drugs.

It is essential that practicing physicians be adequately informed about these issues. However, dosage and precautions specific to the elderly are not commonly found in package inserts, therapeutic texts, and related documents

Table 26.1. Characteristics of the Elderly Physiology

1. Reduced renal function
2. Reduced renin-aldosterone responses
3. Oversecretion of ADH; water intoxication
4. Decreased baroreceptor sensitivity; tendency to orthostatic hypotension
5. Decreased vital capacity and MBC
6. Decreased cardiac output and heart rate response to exercise
7. Large interindividual variations

Table 26.2. Drug Disposition in the Elderly

1. Reduced renal function: Accumulation of renally cleared drugs
2. Reduced serum albumin levels: Increased free drug
3. Relative increase in body fat: Increased Vd of fat-soluble drug
4. Reduction in body size: Decreased Vd of water-soluble drugs
5. Reduction in liver metabolizing capacity: Accumulation of metabolized drugs
6. Increased sensitivity to CNS drugs: Adverse effects
7. Concurrent illnesses: Disease interactions
8. Multiple drugs: Drug interactions
9. Larger interindividual variation: Wide dose range

at present. This follows from the relative infrequency of clinical drug trials designed to measure age-related differences in response to drugs.

In response to the issues noted above, the Food and Drug Administration issued a "discussion paper" for the testing of new drugs in the elderly. This paper has been described in chapter 22. The principal elements are outlined in Table 26.3. A proposal for England enunciated by Professor J. Crooks is outlined in Table 26.4. The "discussion paper" was reviewed by an ad hoc task force on use of drugs in older patients already in place in the Merck organization. The paper and related issues are also being considered by a PMA Medical Section Committee under Dr William Darrow of Schering.

There are substantial areas of agreement between the views of our task force and the FDA discussion paper. The elderly should not be excluded from clinical trials and all drugs should be evaluated for pharmacokinetic properties that might indicate the need for special concern in elderly patients. Appropriate drug interaction studies should be conducted. Much of this activity is part of current practice.

The one area of disagreement is the utility of a pharmacokinetic screening procedure in late Phase II and Phase III trials. Our reservations are listed in Table 26.5. It now appears the concern being proposed by the FDA is much simpler and less "definitive" than the procedure forwarded by Sheiner et al.[5] A true screening procedure to identify individuals or groups whose blood levels differ grossly from the expected, and which is not in itself a measure of efficacy and safety, might be useful. Such a procedure should be tested for utility before being generally recommended. We look forward to discussing this novel approach further with the FDA.

Table 26.3. FDA Discussion Paper

Background
1. Drugs not adequately studied in elderly; included but not analyzed in new drug applications (NDAs)
2. Adverse event incidence and relationship to age unclear
3. Pharmacokinetic changes are related to age but frequency and significance unclear
4. Few documented examples of age-related pharmacodynamic differences

General requirements
1. Formal study of renal excretion with appropriate dosing instructions, including method of estimating creatinine clearance from serum creatinine
2. Evaluate factors that might influence binding of highly bound drugs
3. Implement pharmacokinetic screen in late Phase II and Phase III: described in terms of trough and/or peak sample(s) (intended to detect large interindividual differences)
4. Follow up screen observations
5. Drug interactions: digoxin universal, ophthalmic drugs, hepatic enzyme induction; screen may aid; measure "other" drug levels
6. Disease interactions: include "other" disease(s) in studies; screen may aid

Specific requirements
1. Include elderly in clinical trials of drugs likely to be significantly used in this group
2. Characterize drug actions in the elderly: age, renal/hepatic disease, muscle mass, concomitant therapy and disease, etc
3. Analyze efficacy and safety by age

Table 26.4. The Crooks Proposal for England

Drugs with special problem in elderly:
1. Commonly used in elderly
2. Low Therapeutic ratio and
   a. primary renal elimination
   b. high liver extraction ratio
   c. act on CNS
   d. modified by homeostatic mechanisms impaired in the elderly
Studies proposed, Crooks:
1. Single-dose pharmacokinetic studies in healthy subjects over 70 years of age; multiple-dose studies as needed
2. Pharmacodynamic studies in elderly patients with target disease
3. Establishment of efficacy and safety in elderly under clinical trial conditions using recommended dosing regimen

---

Table 26.5. Pharmacokinetic Screen — Reservations

---

1. Clinical utility unproven for avoiding ADRs or treating individual patients
2. Statistical methodology not validated
   a. Objective criteria for outlier populations
   b. Prospective experience
3. Redundant if efficacy and safety known
4. Unproven practicality
   a. Early, rapid, simple assay procedure
   b. Collection, storage shipment network
   c. Real time assay and interpretation
   d. Double-blind complications
5. Regulatory status of the data

Collecting reliable data on the elderly in the course of controlled clinical trials imposes substantial problems for sponsors, as listed in Table 26.6. We believe the best approach at this time is to focus on drugs whose properties indicate an identifiable hazard for the elderly (Table 26.7). The factors considered are similar to but somewhat broader than those identified by Professor Crooks.

Table 26.6. Problems for Sponsors

1. Populations very heterogeneous
   a. Definitions
   b. Age vs disease vs environment
   c. Ambulatory vs institutional
   d. Multiple drugs
2. Drugs very heterogeneous
   a. Potency/safety ratio
   b. Pharmacokinetic profile
   c. Interaction potential
   d. Metabolites
3. Clinical trials very homogeneous
   a. Design issues
   b. Access to subjects
   c. ADR interpretation and reporting
4. Preparing simple directions from complex data

Table 26.7. Drugs Requiring Special Considerations for Use in Elderly

1. Drugs expected to be widely used in the elderly
2. Drugs that affect or are affected by biologic homeostatic mechanisms that may be deficient in the elderly (eg, the cardiovascular system)
3. Drugs that act in the central nervous system
4. Drugs with a low therapeutic to safety ratio and:
   a. are excreted largely by the kidney
   b. are subject to large first-pass effect
   c. are metabolized by oxidative mechanisms
   d. generate significant metabolites
   e. are highly protein bound

During Phase I and II (Table 26.8), pharmacokinetic (ADME) studies should be conducted in elderly, as well as young, volunteers to identify gross age-related differences and the reasons for the differences, if any. In all phases, elderly who qualify with entrance criteria should be included in clinical trials and the data analyzed for effects of age. Protocols should include pharmacodynamic assessments appropriate to the drug; at a minimum, supine and standing blood pressure and heart rate responses. Early evaluation of links between dose, plasma drug levels, and biologic effect may identify age-related receptor differences and, of course, provide guidance to later studies. If a drug or preparation is targeted for a specific elderly population, we propose that early dose-ranging studies be conducted in this group if at all possible.

Table 26.8. Proposed Approach for the Study of Certain Drugs in the Elderly

---

Phases I and II
1. Early ADME studies in young and elderly subjects
   a. Identify gross age-related differences
   b. Basis of differences, if any
2. Early dose-ranging studies
   a. Include elderly who qualify with entrance criteria
   b. Pharmacodynamic assessment
   c. Link dose, plasma levels and biologic effects
   d. Conduct special studies in target populations for drugs with primary elderly use: glaucoma, parkinsonism, dementia
3. Appropriate drug interaction studies
4. Appropriate disease interaction studies

Phases III to V
1. Include elderly qualifying with entrance criteria; analyze for age-related differences
2. Dedicated studies in appropriate elderly subgroups, such as:
   a. Congestive heart failure
   b. Cardiac arrhythmia
   c. Compromised renal function
   d. Arthritics on NSAIDs
3. A screening method would be useful for the identification of unanticipated hazards

---

Interaction studies with hazardous agents likely to be used concomitantly with the test drug are part of current practice. Such studies need not be conducted in the elderly to provide the requisite information. For less risky drugs, a blood level screening procedure could provide adequate assurance of no clinically significant interaction.

Disease interaction studies could take the form of pharmacokinetic assessments of the effect of renal function, liver function, and protein binding on drug disposition or involve organ function measurements depending on the specific drug and disease under study.

In later phases (Table 26.8), we again propose that elderly qualifying with entrance criteria be admitted to the trials and the results analyzed for age-related differences. When a drug is targeted for a condition common in the elderly, and particularly if the condition is life threatening, a separate study should be conducted to obtain information in elderly patients with the disorder in question.

Finally, for drugs in this category, information gathered during clinical trials in the elderly should be reflected in labeling and other information for health professionals. Drug packages should be easy to open and accompanied by simple, readable instructions for use. Because all of our efforts will be for naught if purveyors and consumers lack requisite information, educational efforts to inform health professionals and consumers about such issues as polypharmacy, the need for accurate reporting by patients, destruction of old unused medications, and the potentially variable response characteristics of elderly patients are essential.

REFERENCES

1. Vestal RE: Aging and pharmacokinetics: Impact of altered physiology in the elderly, in *Physiology and Cell Biology of Aging.* Cherkin A, et al (eds): New York, Raven Press, 1979, pp 185–201.

2. Coe RM: Comprehensive care of the elderly, in Cap RDT, Coe RM, Rossman I (eds): *Fundamentals of Geriatric Medicine.* New York, Raven Press, 1983, pp 3–7.

3. Report of the Royal College of Physicians : Medication for the elderly. *J R Col Physicians* 1984; 18:7–17.

4. Klein LE, German PS and Levine DM: Adverse drug reactions among the elderly: A reassessment. *J Am Geriatr Soc* 1981: 29:525–530.

5. Sheiner LB, Rosenberg B, Marathe VV: Estimation of population characteristics of pharmacokinetic parameters from routine clinical data. *J Pharmacokinet Biopharm* 1977; 5:445–479.

Chapter 27

PATIENT DRUG INFORMATION FOR THE ELDERLY: SOME ONGOING ACTIVITIES

Rhonda B. Friedman, ScD

In 1983, the PMA surveyed its member firms requesting information on all types of patient information distributed to consumers directly or to consumers through the physician. Based on the preliminary analysis of these data, we found that, in 1982, our member firms distributed more than 1,000 different pieces of patient information. Even more impressive than the variety is the reported total number of pieces of information distributed: several hundred million!

More than one third of the 1,000 pieces of material are product specific, with discussions of proper use of medications. About one third of this information is "disease oriented," describing prevention, detection, and treatment of an illness. The remaining information is general in nature, such as tips on keeping fit through exercise or good nutrition.

Not all of these materials are, of course, targeted toward the elderly. While we do know that the elderly use a disproportionate amount of pharmaceuticals in relation to their representation in the population, there is much information produced by our member firms that just wouldn't apply. For example, risks and benefits of childhood immunizations just wouldn't hold the interest of an elderly patient concerned about the side effects of antihypertensive drugs.

Most of the information distributed by pharmaceutical companies is written material (about 71%); another 19% is audiovisual (such as films and cassettes) or visual aids; about 5% is in other forms of media (such as TV and radio); and 4% of all activities are conferences and educational programs.

The majority of the information (59%) is designed to be distributed by the physician to the patient and is not available directly to the public through the company. This is consistent with the industry's view that patient drug information should be delivered by the physician. Nevertheless, 21% of patient information materials are available to the consumer directly — most of this information, though, is disease or general health oriented, not product specific.

It is very difficult to determine which of these materials is developed for use by the elderly alone and which others are targeted at all patients. It is clear, though, that our companies produce information on products in every therapeutic class used by elderly patients. Some of these categories include analgesics and antiarthritics, anticoagulants, antiinfective agents, antiparkinsonians, bronchial agents, anticancer drugs, cardiovascular drugs, diuretics, ophthalmics, and psychotherapeutic agents. In addition, information on menopause, osteoporosis, pneumococcal pneumonia, and general health information on growing older is made available to elderly consumers. Also, special pains are taken to use large type, etc, for easy reading and comprehension.

Perhaps the two best known company-sponsored education projects for the elderly are the "Elder Ed" program (Parke-Davis) and the "Med Ed" program (Roche Laboratories). The Elder Ed program is sponsored through a grant to the University of Maryland School of Pharmacy in Baltimore. The Maryland Pharmaceutical Association also is involved. The program utilizes retired pharmacist volunteers to present drug compliance information to other elders. A similar program, sponsored by Roche, is implemented through Rutgers University. Their program also urges pharmacy students to go out and speak to senior citizen groups.

These programs have been great successes. In addition, Parke-Davis had implemented a poster/pamphlet program through participating pharmacies urging elderly patients to ask their pharmacists about the drugs that have been prescribed. The programs are going strong and there are plans for expansion.

We have seen that hundreds of millions of materials were distributed in 1982 to patients and that the elderly have been targeted for much of this information. About 60% of the materials are distributed through physicians and pharmacists. We know that hundreds of millions of pieces of materials were given to health professionals for distribution, but is that information filtering down to the patient? The answer is: We really don't know.

An FDA study last year suggests that consumers do not remember receiving such information from their physician or pharmacist. We believe that the responsibility for improving this communication lies both with the patient and the physician. That is why the "Get the Answers" campaign promoted by the National Council on Patient Information and Education (NCPIE) is so important. Our survey tells us that the physicians have the materials, but the patients need to be motivated to ask for them and the doctors need to be motivated to use them. Experience with the AMA program suggests that special efforts need to be made to motivate physicians.

Another FDA survey undertaken last year reported that about 20% of doctors use pamphlets produced by pharmaceutical companies on a weekly basis. This confirms our sense that the pamphlets are useful. But why aren't more physicians using these readily available materials? How can we sensitize and motivate a busy physician in a hectic office practice to take the time to educate patients? Physicians need to be motivated to "Give the Answers." With the excellent program sponsored by the AMA, the excellent efforts of NCPIE, and the multitude of materials available through the industry, this should be an attainable goal. It is not a lack of information that impedes the transfer of knowledge. And the availability of information alone will not assure proper use of drugs, either prescribed by the doctor or used by the patient.

Physicians and consumers need to be made aware of these materials or motivated to use them. We believe we have made a good start. We urge you to take advantage of these resources.

PART 11

THE FUTURE IN GERIATRIC DRUG USE

Chapter 28

THE IMPORTANCE OF DRUG USE AS AN ISSUE FOR THE ELDERLY

Ike Andrews

As a layman whose job brings me into contact with a great many facets of the health problems of the aging, I want to discuss what I have read and heard that led me to introduce legislation that I hope will result in improved health education programs for older Americans.

First of all, I have been deeply involved with the issues of aging since I came to Congress in 1972. As a charter member of the Select Aging Committee and ranking member of that Committee's Health and Long Term Care Subcommittee, I have taken part in hearings on just about every aspect of health and the elderly. I am also chairman of the Education and Labor Subcommittee on Human Resources, which has jurisdiction over the Older Americans Act, the major federal initiative for the elderly. I wrote the reauthorization of that Act in 1981 and have just introduced legislation to extend its program for an additional 3 years.

During the fall of 1983, some factors came together for me. On one hand, the health of my own mother, who is now 84 years old, was increasingly on my mind. In addition, as reauthorization approached, my staff and I have been studying the results of the 1981 White House Conference on Aging to determine what advice we could glean in preparation for the reauthorization bill. One group of recommendations that occurred in a number of places in the conference reports caught my eye. These have to do with "wellness," the promotion of "wellness," and the role of health education and self-care in that connection.

Let me quote from the conference's final report:

Recommendation: . . . The Federal Government should provide financial support for the development of nationwide demonstration projects in geriatric health promotion which include all the elements of the wellness approach: self-responsibility, physical fitness, stress management, and nutrition and environmental awareness.

The conference's Committee on the Promotion and Maintenance of Wellness specifically addressed the drug issue by recommending:

> The elderly should be educated in the safe and effective use of prescription medicines.

We know that drugs have a great impact on all our lives, but their effect on the elderly is greatly magnified. According to statistics from the Department of Health and Human Services, four out of five Americans over 65 years of age suffer from one or more chronic health problems. In most cases this results in frequent medication, either self-prescribed or physician-prescribed. And in many cases, the medication alone, or in combination with attention to such things as exercise and nutrition, makes it possible for the great majority of these people to live normal, active lives. So drugs can be of great importance to the "quality of life" for an older person.

At a hearing on "Drug Use and Misuse Among Older Americans," held in June 1983, by the Select Aging Committee, we heard that Americans over 65, representing some 11% of the population, consume about one-third of the prescriptions written annually, or about 13 prescriptions per year for each individual in that age group. Add to that the large number of nonprescription drugs taken by the elderly and one gets a clear picture of the potential for harmful interaction of the various drugs an individual might be taking at a given time.

At that same hearing, a witness from a Florida drug information center told about ten years' experience in talking with older clients who had drug-related concerns. His list included:

- drug interactions — what happens when the amount prescribed may be too much, or the patient decides for himself or herself that, if a little bit is good, more is better

- self-medication — individuals decide whether or not to take a prescribed drug, for a variety of reasons — including economic

- outdated drugs — retaining unused prescriptions and self-prescribing them at a considerably later date

- automatic refills — misuse of refill provisions, with inadequate supervision from a physician

- confusion — in very elderly patients, particularly if several drugs are being prescribed simultaneously

- tamperproof packaging — childproof sometimes means patient-proof too

This list can be expanded, as we all know. In thinking about the problem of drug misuse, overuse, and underuse, it has seemed to me that the place where the necessary information and concern and awareness can all come together is not in any one professional but in the older persons themselves. And that belief led me to look at ways to do a better job of providing information and education programs for those most involved with improving the health of older Americans — the older Americans themselves.

As I mentioned, one of the pieces of legislation under my subcommittee's jurisdiction is the Older Americans Act, and I have come to believe that part of the answer to better health information and education for older people can be found in the structure presently existing under that act.

Some 3,300 senior citizens centers have been established throughout the country, with one or more in nearly every city and town. Millions of older Americans gather at these centers each day — more than 9 million during last year. In addition, as I have learned through the School of Public Health at the University of North Carolina at Chapel Hill, there are 23 graduate schools of public health around the country, with approximately 1,700 faculty members and some 9,000 students.

The bill I have introduced, HR 4472, will bring these two great public activities — the Older Americans Act and the schools of public health, and possibly other institutions of higher learning — together for the advantage and enhancement of both. HR 4472 would establish a new title to the Older Americans Act, Title VII, to add health education and training to the services already provided to senior citizens who participate in the Older Americans Act programs. It will provide for the use of senior centers as classrooms, the leadership of schools of public health as curriculum developers, and the 9 million or so center participants as students. It is my intention to do all I can to see that this bill is signed into law as part of the Older Americans Act.

My bill is certainly not the whole answer, nor is it wholly new. But I view it as a step forward in an effort to make these last years, these years that are increasing as medical science extends our life expectancy, more active, more meaningful, and more "in control."

I hope that everyone reading this chapter is able to join us in this important effort on behalf of our older Americans. Because we are all aging, drug education as well as health education is vital to each of us.

Chapter 29

THE FUTURE AND GERIATRIC DRUG USE

Clement Bezold, PhD

We often extend what we know, what we are familiar with, into the future, only to be surprised that the future does not turn out to be quite like the past. The future of drug use, particularly in the elderly, is likely to be in that category.

In thinking about the future of geriatric drug use, there are some issues that relate to the future of drugs, some to the future of drug use monitoring, and some that relate to larger questions about approaches to health care. One way to simultaneously consider an array of divergent possibilities is to create scenarios. These scenarios or alternative futures present divergent "future histories" against which to consider today's decisions. (For more information on alternative futures for health care, see the article "Health Care in the United States: Four alternative futures" in the August 1982, issue of *The Futurist*.)

I will restrict my remarks to two of the areas that will affect geriatric drug use. The first is the future of pharmaceuticals and the second is the future of computers in health care and their application to the monitoring of drug use (as well as monitoring other therapeutic approaches).

Much of the concern over drug use by the elderly comes from the situations of multiple prescriptions for the same patient sometimes without adequate concern for drug interactions, emphasis on drug therapy over other therapies because of the absence of training or support for nutrition or other health promotion or self-care approaches, and a general lack of certainty about the effects of drugs on the elderly because of their virtual absence from the pools of subjects in the clinical trials that established the drug's safety and efficacy in the first place. This book has reviewed the diverse approaches to overcoming these problems and they need the serious attention this book reflects. Yet the future may provide some interesting solutions to some of today's problems.

THE FUTURE OF PHARMACEUTICALS

Part of the problem in current drug therapy is that many drugs are what Lewis Thomas and Burton Weisbrod have described as "half-way technologies." Unable to prevent or cure the disease, they work to ameliorate the symptoms. Moreover, the therapeutic specificity of drugs is increasingly more focused. Many problems stem from the need to bathe the entire body, usually through the bloodstream, with the toxic chemical in the drug. The years ahead may see much more sophisticated, and much more precisely targeted, pharmaceuticals. The prospects in this area have led Thomas to argue that diseases are biological puzzles that we are on the verge of solving.

Science and medical writers Jane Stein and William Check have surveyed leading academic, government, and industry researchers on the prospects for new drugs in the years ahead, and have reported in *Pharmaceuticals in the Year 2000* and *Pharmacy in the 21st Century*. Stein's and Check's surveys found that a variety of experts have speculated that within two or three decades we may have effective drugs or vaccines to prevent most cancers, to prevent various viral diseases, and to treat autoimmune diseases.

Pharmaceutical R&D has moved the target of drugs from the whole body to organ systems and then to specific cells. In the future, drugs might be targeted to specific subcellular parts. Take anticancer drugs in the future. We are learning about the genetic switches — the oncogenes — that make a normal cell become malignant. It is now suspected that there are antioncogenes that keep the oncogenes from being expressed. Once the antioncogenes are discovered it may be possible to seed these antioncogenes throughout the body via a deactivated virus.

Alternatively, for those suffering from cancer, monoclonal antibodies will provide more targeted therapy. Current cell-killing drugs attack all growing cells in the body. Future therapies will be able to target cancer cells. Thus a distinctive antigen, which appears only on the surface of the cancer cells, can become the target for a specially developed monoclonal antibody. This more focused therapy would avoid the gastrointestinal and other side effects of current cancer drugs. The same monoclonal antibodies might also be used as the carriers of more toxic chemicals, releasing their cargo only when the antibody was bound to the proper cell.

Neurotransmitter research may yield a cure for Alzheimer's disease and identify more potent pharmocological agents for depression and other mental conditions. This research may also tell how each of us through our diet, exercise, and biofeedback or other "mental exercises" can increase the appropriate brain chemicals to calm us or to lift us out of depression.

COMPUTERS AND HEALTH CARE

Computers, software programs, and human networks using the two together may have profound effects on health care and on drug use. Health care is an information industry. Physicians develop a knowledge base, or an awareness of where to find knowledge, and a set of clinical practice algorithms that direct their judgment. Already, leading clinicians in various fields have teamed up with computer experts to put their "decision-tree" into computer programs. One of these, CADUSEUS, deals with problems of internal medicine and will diagnose better than a general practitioner and will compete with specialists in internal medicine. In the years ahead these diagnostic programs will become more sophisticated and cover more than single fields of medicine.

Computerization of medical record keeping, through programs such as the PROMIS system developed by Dr Lawrence Weed, will make medical management much better aware of what is happening to patients. Combine this with the pressures surrounding prospective payment programs for hospitals using diagnostic-related groups (DRGs) and you have a variety of pressures for the providers and the funders of the health care system to become much better managers.

At the same time, consumers are entering the field, seeking computer programs for health promotion, and they are joining together to scrutinize health care providers. Market research firms see impressive growth for the sales of health-related software to consumers interested in health promotion. Consumer groups, such as the People's Medical Society, are developing sophisticated projects to monitor local hospital and other health care providers (much as business coalitions in various cities throughout the country).

What will this mean for drug use and the elderly? The more targeted drugs should mean few side effects. The use of health monitoring programs by consumers can provide the person's own biochemically unique profile (built up over a period of time) so that he or she can closely monitor the effects of single or multiple prescriptions. At the same time, we will be better able to do "prospective epidemiology" and identify which individuals are at the greatest risk of side effects to particular drugs.

Groups of consumers will monitor drug effects via computer conferencing and electronic networks, even as informal discussion groups of physicians and pharmacists on computer networks now do. (These groups spotted and shared information on side effect problems of one drug recently removed from the market, and did so ahead of the FDA.) In the years ahead, groups such as AARP or the Health Research Group are likely to form monitoring systems of various kinds using these emerging technologies. Although these will not immediately supplant the need for regulation by the FDA, they will be able to provide consumers, including the elderly, with more rapid, sophisticated, and organized input into the pharmaceutical marketplace. The FDA and other government agencies interested in or responsible for monitoring drug use should encourage these efforts and work to ensure that they are as comparable as possible, given their unfunded and voluntary effort, to other more official postmarketing monitoring changes.

All in all, drugs will be an important part of the elderly life study in the next century — either having prevented the onset of some diseases or treating in more targeted ways those diseases that do occur.

Chapter 30

MOVING FORWARD IN THE GERIATRIC DRUG AREA — A SUMMATION

Daniel D. Cowell, MD

The changing demographics of aging with which you are well-acquainted represents a stunning triumph of survivorship, attributable in part to medical technology and the environmental sciences. But this great achievement — permitting even more people to live out their God-given life spans, carries with it the responsibility to provide for their safety, economic sufficiency, housing, nutrition, and especially, health care. Therefore there is a need for new knowledge and skills on the part of physicians, nurses, dentists, pharmacists and other care givers who serve the elderly.

Several points in this regard are worth noting: (1) the placing of geriatrics-related material on professional Board and licensure examinations might stimulate the professions to take greater interest in the elderly; (2) there needs to be more emphasis upon building the capacity for geriatric medicine, dentistry and nursing in professional schools — the NIA has done this in the case of medical schools via 26 Geriatric Medicine Academic Awards it has made; (3) the process of obtaining informed consent from the patient before prescribing patient neuroleptic medication common to the practice of psychiatry, may spread to other areas of medicine, creating more informed providers as well as consumers; (4) and finally, the profession of pharmacy may yet provide the leadership to help guide other professions out of the present prescribing problems involving the elderly, by being the focal point and repository of information about a given patient's drug profile.

Related to factors on drug interactions, one factor that is often related to non-compliance that we know about, yet tend to overlook, is that of the cost to the patient of polypharmacy and complex drug regimens. Many patients simply cannot afford — or believe they cannot afford — medication as prescribed. It is important, when possible, to use generic forms, prescribe larger tablet sizes, and to advise the patient that they can have a portion of the prescription filled at one time and the remainder when needed.

The helping professions need to do more with respect to education of the public about prescription and non-prescription drugs. Unless this is done, the national media will continue to serve as a source of such information, eg, the recent television report by a noted journalist involving tardive dyskinesia, which probably unduly alarmed many patients who really need to take neuroleptic medication on a regular basis.

In summation, today's older person has been raised to regard the doctor's word as gospel and his authority in medical matters as unchallengeable. Yet, these same older people may still harbor private reservations about the prescriptions they have been given whether related to cost, the tone and quality of the encounter with the doctor, his perceived level of interest, the inconvenience entailed in complying with treatment, awareness of drug side effects, or for other reasons. To the extent this is so, I think older patients make their own independent evaluation of the care they have received, but do not bring themselves to take open issue with the physician, often so as not to "hurt the doctor's feelings." Tomorrow's elderly, ie, today's youth, should be better educated about the uses, abuses, and misues of medication as the cohort's orientation toward physician's (and toward authority in general) will probably be quite different in their old age, than what we know is characteristic of today's elderly.

ABOUT THE EDITORS AND CONTRIBUTORS

The Editors

Steven R. Moore MPH is a pharmacist with the Office of Drug Standards, Food and Drug Administration in Rockville, MD. He also serves on the Public Health Service/Administration on Aging Task Group on Health Promotion for the Elderly, and serves as Senior Advisor on Geriatric Drugs to the Office of Disease Prevention and Health Promotion (DHHS). His address is Food and Drug Administration, 5600 Fishers Lane, Rockville, MD 20857

Mr Thomas W. Teal is the Director of Scientific Data Management, McNeil Pharmaceutical; the Administrative Director of the Drug Information Association; and Editor-in-Chief, Drug Information Journal. His address is PO Box 113, Maple Glen, PA 19002

The Contributors

C. Everett Koop, MD is the Surgeon General, US Public Health Service Deputy Assistant Secretary for Health, US Department of Health and Human Services. His address is Room 18-16, PHS, 5600 Fishers Lane, Rockville, MD 20857

Lennie-Marie P. Tolliver, PhD is the US Commissioner on Aging. Her address is Room 4760, HHHS, 330 Independence Ave SW, Washington, DC 20201

Lloyd G. Millstein, PhD is the Director, Drug Advertising and Labeling, Food and Drug Administration. His address is HFN-240, 5600 Fishers Lane, Rockville, MD 20857

Nancy J. Olins, MA is with the American Association of Retired Persons, Pharmacy Service. Her address is 510 King St, Suite 420, Alexandria, VA 22314

Kenneth F. Lampe, PhD is with the Division of Drugs and Technology, American Medical Association, Chicago, IL 60610

Albert G. Eckian, MD is the Medical and Scientific Consultant for the Proprietary Association. His address is 242 Lincolnshire Rd, Winter Park, FL 32792

Robert E. Vestal, MD is Chief, Geriatric Clinical Pharmacology Unit, Director, Research Program, Veterans Administration Medical Center, Boise, ID 83702 and Associate Profesor of Medicine, University of Washington School of Medicine, Seattle, WA 83702

Robert E. Allen, PhD is the Special Assistant to the Director, Medical Research Service, Veterans Administration Central Office, Washington, DC 20420

George M. Steinberg is with the Pharmacology Program, Geriatrics Branch, Room 5C15A, Bldg 31, NIA/NIH, Bethesda, MD 20205

Daniel A. Hussar, PhD is the Dean of Faculty and Remington Professor of Pharmacy at the Philadelphia College of Pharmacy. His address is 43rd St and King Sessing Mall, Philadelphia, PA 19104

B. Robert Meyer, MD is the Chief, Division of Clinical Pharmacology, North Shore Univeristy Hospital, Manhasset, NY 11030

Dr M.N. Graham Dukes, is the Regional Officer for Pharmaceuticals, World Health Organization. His address is Regional Office for Europe, Copenhagen, Denmark.

T. Franklin Williams, MD is the Director, National Institute on Aging, National Institutes of Health. His address is Room 2C05, Building 31, NIA/NIH, Bethesda, MD 20205

Carlene Baum, PhD, **Dianne L. Kennedy,** RPh, MPH, and **Mary B. Forbes,** RPh are with the Drug Use Analysis Branch, National Center for Drugs and Biologics, Food and Drug Administration. Their address is 5600 Fishers Lane, Rockville, MD 20857

Judith K. Jones, MD, PhD, is with the Division of Drug and Biological Product Experience, Food and Drug Administration. Her address is 5600 Fishers Lane, Rockville, MD 20857

Robert B. Wallace, MD is with the Department of Preventive Medicine and Environmental Health, University of Iowa, Iowa City, IA 52242

Jerry Avorn, MD is the Assistant Professor of Social Medicine and Health Policy and the Director, Drug Information Program of the Harvard Medical School. His address is 643 Huntington Ave, Boston, MA 02115

Fred Wegner is with the American Association of Retired Persons. His address is 1909 K St NW, Washington, DC 20037

Mary S. Harper, PhD, RN, FAAN is the Coordinator, Long Term Care Programs. Her address is Room 11C03, NIMH, 5600 Fishers Lane, Rockville, MD 20857

Marion J. Finkel, MD is the Director, Office of Orphan Products Development. Her address is HF-35/FDA, 5600 Fishers Lane, Rockville, MD 20857

David J. Greenblatt, MD is the Chief, Division of Clinical Pharmacology, Professor of Psychiatry and Associate Professor of Medicine, Tufts-New England Medical Center, Boston, MA 02111

Darrell P. Abernethy, MD, PhD is the Assistant Profesor of Medicine at the Baylor College of Medicine in Houston, TX 77030

Richard I. Shader, MD is the Professor and Chairman, Department of Psychiatry Tufts-New England Medical Center, Boston, MA 02111

Robert Straus, PhD is Professor and Chairman, Department of Behavioral Science, College of Medicine, at the University of Kentucky, Lexington, KY 40536

Robert Temple, MD is the Director, Office of Drug Research and Review, National Center for Drugs and Biologics, HFN-100, Food and Drug Administration, 5600 Fishers Lane, Rockville, MD 20857

Frances O. Kelsey, PhD, MD is the Director, Division of Scientific Investigations, HFN-220, Food and Drug Administration, 5600 Fishers Lane, Rockville, MD 20857

J. Michael McGinnis, MD is the Deputy Assistant Secretary for Health, US Department of Health and Human Services. His address is Room 719-H, 200 Independence Ave SW, Washington, DC 20201

Hugh H. Tilson, MD, Dr PH is the Director, Product Surveillance and Epidemiology at the Burroughs Wellcome Co. His address is Research Triangle Park, NC 27709

William B. Abrams, MD is the Executive Director of Scientific Development at Merck & Co, West Point, PA 19486

Rhonda B. Friedman, ScD is the Senior Analyst, Pharmaceutical Manufacturers Association. Her address is 1155 15th St NW, Washington, DC 20005

Representative Ike Andrews (D-NC) is the Chairman, Subcommittee on Human Resources, House Committee on Education and Labor, US House of Representatives, Washington, DC 20515

Clement Bezold, PhD is the Executive Director, Institute for Alternative Futures. His address is 1624 Cresent Pl NW, Washington, DC 22313.

Daniel D. Cowell, MD is Associate Director for Medical Education, National Institute of Health Clinical Center, Bethesda, MD 20850.